Philippa Pigache has been a journalist and writer for more than thirty years, starting on local newspapers and women's magazines, moving to national newspapers, radio and television and, more recently, becoming a freelance medical science writer. She has worked on the *Sunday Times*, *Daily Mail* and *Guardian*, and for ITN and BBC science features.

She started to specialize in writing about medicine chiefly because she was married to a doctor. (Her own educational background is in modern languages and the theatre.) She has contributed to consumer health pages and journals for health professionals for twenty years and has won awards for her medical journalism and also for her fiction. She is currently the honorary secretary of the Medical Journalists' Association and editor of their journal, the *MJA News*.

She has written consumer health books on lupus, arthritis and Attention Deficit Hyperactivity Disorder (ADHD). Her first book for Sheldon Press, *Living with Rheumatoid Arthritis*, was commended in the 2005 MJA Open Consumer Book Awards. She has two children, three grandchildren and three cats. She lives in Sussex and paints and gardens in her spare time.

_he
to r
www
www

Overcoming Common Problems Series

Selected titles

A full list of titles is available from Sheldon Press,
36 Causton Street, London SW1P 4ST, and on our website at
www.sheldonpress.co.uk

Assertiveness: Step by Step
Dr Windy Dryden and Daniel Constantinou

Breaking Free
Carolyn Ainscough and Kay Toon

Calm Down
Paul Hauck

Cataract: What You Need to Know
Mark Watts

Cider Vinegar
Margaret Hills

Comfort for Depression
Janet Horwood

Confidence Works
Gladeana McMahon

Coping Successfully with Pain
Neville Shone

Coping Successfully with Panic Attacks
Shirley Trickett

Coping Successfully with Period Problems
Mary-Claire Mason

Coping Successfully with Prostate Cancer
Dr Tom Smith

Coping Successfully with Ulcerative Colitis
Peter Cartwright

Coping Successfully with your Hiatus Hernia
Dr Tom Smith

Coping Successfully with Your Irritable Bowel
Rosemary Nicol

Coping with Alopecia
Dr Nigel Hunt and Dr Sue McHale

Coping with Anxiety and Depression
Shirley Trickett

Coping with Blushing
Dr Robert Edelmann

Coping with Bowel Cancer
Dr Tom Smith

Coping with Brain Injury
Maggie Rich

Coping with Candida
Shirley Trickett

Coping with Chemotherapy
Dr Terry Priestman

Coping with Childhood Allergies
Jill Eckersley

Coping with Childhood Asthma
Jill Eckersley

Coping with Chronic Fatigue
Trudie Chalder

Coping with Coeliac Disease
Karen Brody

Coping with Cystitis
Caroline Clayton

Coping with Depression and Elation
Patrick McKeon

Coping with Down's Syndrome
Fiona Marshall

Coping with Dyspraxia
Jill Eckersley

Coping with Eating Disorders and Body Image
Christine Craggs-Hinton

Coping with Eczema
Dr Robert Youngson

Coping with Endometriosis
Jo Mears

Coping with Epilepsy
Fiona Marshall and Dr Pamela Crawford

Coping with Fibroids
Mary-Claire Mason

Coping with Gout
Christine Craggs-Hinton

Coping with Heartburn and Reflux
Dr Tom Smith

Coping with Incontinence
Dr Joan Gomez

Coping with Long-Term Illness
Barbara Baker

Coping with Macular Degeneration
Dr Patricia Gilbert

Coping with the Menopause
Janet Horwood

Overcoming Common Problems Series

Coping with a Mid-Life Crisis
Derek Milne

Coping with Polycystic Ovary Syndrome
Christine Craggs-Hinton

Coping with Postnatal Depression
Sandra L. Wheatley

Coping with SAD
Fiona Marshall and Peter Cheevers

Coping with Snoring and Sleep Apnoea
Jill Eckersley

Coping with a Stressed Nervous System
Dr Kenneth Hambly and Alice Muir

Coping with Strokes
Dr Tom Smith

Coping with Suicide
Maggie Helen

Coping with Thyroid Problems
Dr Joan Gomez

Depression
Dr Paul Hauck

Depression at Work
Vicky Maud

Depressive Illness
Dr Tim Cantopher

Eating for a Healthy Heart
Robert Povey, Jacqui Morrell and Rachel Povey

Effortless Exercise
Dr Caroline Shreeve

Fertility
Julie Reid

Free Your Life from Fear
Jenny Hare

Getting a Good Night's Sleep
Fiona Johnston

Heal the Hurt: How to Forgive and Move On
Dr Ann Macaskill

Heart Attacks – Prevent and Survive
Dr Tom Smith

Help Your Child Get Fit Not Fat
Jan Hurst and Sue Hubberstey

Helping Children Cope with Anxiety
Jill Eckersley

Helping Children Cope with Change and Loss
Rosemary Wells

Helping Children Get the Most from School
Sarah Lawson

How to Be Your Own Best Friend
Dr Paul Hauck

How to Beat Pain
Christine Craggs-Hinton

How to Cope with Bulimia
Dr Joan Gomez

How to Cope with Difficult People
Alan Houel and Christian Godefroy

How to Improve Your Confidence
Dr Kenneth Hambly

How to Keep Your Cholesterol in Check
Dr Robert Povey

How to Stick to a Diet
Deborah Steinberg and Dr Windy Dryden

How to Stop Worrying
Dr Frank Tallis

Hysterectomy
Suzie Hayman

Is HRT Right for You?
Dr Anne MacGregor

Letting Go of Anxiety and Depression
Dr Windy Dryden

Lifting Depression the Balanced Way
Dr Lindsay Corrie

Living with Alzheimer's Disease
Dr Tom Smith

Living with Asperger Syndrome
Dr Joan Gomez

Living with Asthma
Dr Robert Youngson

Living with Autism
Fiona Marshall

Living with Crohn's Disease
Dr Joan Gomez

Living with Diabetes
Dr Joan Gomez

Living with Fibromyalgia
Christine Craggs-Hinton

Living with Food Intolerance
Alex Gazzola

Living with Grief
Dr Tony Lake

Overcoming Common Problems Series

Overcoming Common Problems

How to be a Healthy Weight

PHILIPPA PIGACHE

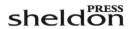

First published in Great Britain in 2007

Sheldon Press
36 Causton Street
London SW1P 4ST

British Library Cataloguing-in-Publication Data
A catalogue record for this book is available from the British Library

ISBN-13: 978–0–85969–981–5

1 3 5 7 9 10 8 6 4 2

Typeset by Northern Phototypesetting Co Ltd, Bolton
Printed in Great Britain by Ashford Colour Press, Hampshire

Contents

To Andrew

with whom I eat, exercise and cultivate our garden

Introduction

One of the great ironies of the twenty-first century is that while a mass of people in the developing world struggle with poverty and hunger, those in the developed nations continually try to eat less and lose weight. Surveys reveal that at any one time as many as three-quarters of the population of the United Kingdom or the United States are on some kind of diet. At some time or other 90 per cent have tried to lose weight. Weight-loss treatments and foods amount to a $50 billion a year business. 'One billion people overweight worldwide,' scream the headlines; overweight and obesity cause 400,000 premature deaths in the USA alone, we are told. Apparently food and drink, fundamental human needs, are killing us.

It was not always so. Scarcely 200 years ago, curves that went out as well as in were regarded as an essential part of femininity, and a generous 'corporation' straining at the waistcoat buttons was a badge of manly maturity. Historically, people linked thinness with poverty and illness, and bulk (what you and I call 'fat') with wealth, vitality and female beauty. It's a link that is still made in parts of Africa and South America. The wives of the king of Uganda were encouraged to become so fat they could scarcely stand. It demonstrated that he was so rich they didn't need to: he could afford to have them carried everywhere.

But somewhere in the first half of the twentieth century, curves went out of fashion. A vogue for adolescent slimness took their place. In the second half of that century, medical experts reinforced the new aesthetic: being fat, we learned, was unhealthy. Bit by bit, the charge list against being fat stacked up: it made you more susceptible to osteoarthritis, high blood pressure, high *cholesterol*, heart disease, *diabetes* . . . the list went on. Fat fear ruled, and still does.

This book is designed to help you achieve a balance in this climate of fear: to sort the good sense from the hype, and to make informed decisions about your weight. Being overweight is not an illness. Nor is obesity, despite what you may have read, although it may increase your risk of disease. This is not a diet book, though inevitably it will look at the many diets that assail us in the pages of newspapers, magazines and other slim volumes like this. My goal is to explore the proven health implications of being heavy or fat *and* underweight; to expose the unsubstantiated scare stories; and to look at what makes people heavy in the first place and, if you do decide you need to lose weight, what choices are open to you.

Who is overweight anyway; who obese? How is it calculated? Should you be pursuing an ideal weight or trying to find out what's right for you? All the evidence points to our not being designed to be identical in body weight and shape, so *vive la différence!* It doesn't mean we can't be healthy and happy with what we have. Ultimately, I hope that reading this book will enable you to go back into the bathroom and face the scales with a light heart – or, better still, chuck them in the bin.

Hints on reading this book

The subject of weight and health is a banquet of gargantuan proportions. I have tried to reduce it to the size of a light lunch and make it as digestible as possible. There is quite a lot of science in it and a sprinkling of history, but served in small helpings, attractively presented. I've designed it so that you can take the full menu, nibble a bit here or there or skip a whole course if you feel full.

In the first four chapters I review the science that connects health and weight. Chapter 1 asks what it means to call someone fat, heavy or overweight, and how it was that being overweight came to be seen as unattractive, unhealthy or even sinful. I look at how a healthy body weight has been calculated – from mortality figures to the dreaded body-mass index (BMI). We also look at how the physical constituents of your body – muscle and bone as well as fat – and their distribution, contribute to your weight and your health. I recommend you read this chapter although it is long because understanding how obesity and overweight are calculated makes you better able to evaluate reports on the health risks associated with weight, or shape for that matter. Chapter 2 looks at the factors that determine how much someone weighs – build, genes, experience before birth or in childhood, physical activity and environmental factors like eating behaviour. Chapter 3 looks in more detail at the health risks, including the risk of joint damage and type 2 (non insulin dependent) diabetes, two of the conditions most clearly linked to excess weight, but also identifies when fat reserves are positively beneficial and dieting risky. Chapter 4 looks at slimming diets and their history, different sorts of diet and particularly the awful see-saw of yo-yo dieting, as well as diet pills and more extreme measures involving surgery.

The second part of the book considers ways in which you can influence the balance between health and weight. Chapter 5 looks at how habits and factors influencing the *metabolism* may occur in early life or even in the womb. Chapter 6 discusses how you may successfully go about avoiding or limiting weight gain, including the importance of changing your relationship to food, having a good body image and not teaching yourself to accept failure. Chapter 7 outlines the healthy, happy diet: both eating for health and dieting to reduce weight. Chapter 8 looks at the importance of exercise – how much and what sort, and how it influences your weight and your well-being. Finally, Chapter 9 looks at life-goals you set yourself; not only being healthy and maybe a certain weight, but being happy and fulfilled and at peace with yourself: what the French call *être bien dans sa peau*, to be happy in your own skin. Because this, we sincerely believe, is what it really means to be fit, or fit for life. Weight and fat are the smallest part of fitness; being active, balanced and positive matter ten times more.

Throughout the book, cross-headings and titles will help you find your way around, skip what you want, and zero in on what concerns you. Difficult words are explained in the text and those printed in *italic type* when they first appear (though not throughout the text) are listed in the glossary at the end of the book. Interesting information is picked out in separate boxes. Finally, don't overlook the section on further reading (p. 115), which contains details of the books and articles mentioned, and the useful addresses (p. 107).

*A healthy weight is the weight a person maintains
while living a healthy life.*
(Paul Campos, The Obesity Myth)

*A woman shouldn't be skinny or fat. She should be the size
that is natural to her. Women are all different but all women
can be beautiful.*
(Giuseppe Miroglio, Italian fashion designer,
whose label caters for women ranging from size 12 to 26)

Part 1

WEIGHING UP THE EVIDENCE

1

Who are you calling overweight?

Worried about weight or body fat? Restore your sense of proportion by looking at *The Judgement of Paris* by Peter Paul Rubens in London's National Gallery. Better still, go to the library and look up the Willendorf Venus. (Or visit: <http://employees.oneonta.edu/angellkg/prehist.html>.) Slim waifs these goddesses are not. And yet they represented the ideal of beauty, vitality, femininity in its prime as viewed by generations since pre-history.

The ideal body shape has varied according to time and place. In terms of geography, people the world over tend to admire a body shape close to that of the average healthy local individual in the prime of life – small and dark in Japan, tall and fair in Scandinavia. Throughout history, however, the fashionable ideal has morphed, and ordinary women (or rich women, at any rate), and sometimes men too, have attempted to modify their figures, corseting the waist, padding the hips, even strapping down the breasts in the 1920s. Being fat and thin in the right places has been the goal of the fashion-conscious rich for centuries, but it wasn't until the eighteenth century that a connection emerged between being overweight and illness. In the succeeding 250 years something really weird has happened. The ideal body has become so ultra slim that models in Western fashion magazines today resemble not healthy adults so much as immature adolescents with an eating disorder. This particular idealized body shape is so remote from the norm that the real-life woman on a Clapham omnibus strives in vain to get anywhere near it.

So how is it that overweight and body fat have come to be regarded as serious health hazards, while an emaciated ideal, sometimes called 'heroin chic', queens it on the front page of *Vogue*? For centuries everyone regarded thinness, or losing weight (wasting, as occurred in tuberculosis), as the mark of sickness. Even today, doctors taking a medical history will ask, 'Have you lost weight?' They may also ask you if you've gained weight, because any extreme or sudden changes in body weight are now recognized as symptoms of illness. Some 300 years ago, when food supplies were unreliable, not on tap at the nearest supermarket, storing body fat conferred major survival advantages.

Shakespeare was in no doubt that bulk was admirable in a man: 'A goodly portly man, i'faith, and a corpulent one,' he says of Falstaff in *Henry IV*, and as late as the end of the nineteenth century, women like the American feminist Elizabeth Cadey Standon were praised for a 'mature' figure. Studies of painted portraits (mostly, it is true, of the well-off) reveal a steady growth in corpulence, especially in those over 40, from Shakespeare's time until the end of the eighteenth century, after which it starts to decline – until the late twentieth century, since when, we are constantly reminded, it has started to rise again. It is probably not a coincidence that the long decline in the rate of corpulence in the upper classes was associated with increased medical understanding of the link between overweight and illness.

Early 'fat' doctors

Way ahead of his time, an eighteenth-century Italian physician called Morgagni noticed from post-mortems that a particular form of fat distribution – the sort that builds up outside round the stomach and internally around major body organs – was associated with high blood pressure, the build-up of fatty deposits in blood vessels known as *atheroma* (one of the warning signs of heart disease), blood abnormalities that suggested the kidneys were not working well, and a tendency to *obstructive sleep apnoea* (OSA) – a potentially fatal event when someone, usually snoring, stops breathing abruptly during sleep, and may die. In early eighteenth-century England, a physician called George Cheyne, who struggled with his weight all his life – on one occasion he ballooned to a massive 450 pounds (205 kilos) – blamed the increasing phenomenon of obesity among the upper classes upon new wealth, sedentary habits and city living. (Sounds familiar?) (A short history of slimming appears in Chapter 4, pp. 40–3.)

By the end of the century (1780) a Scottish physician called Flemyng made a keen observation: weight gain became hazardous to health only when it became so extreme that it prevented activity and bodily function. 'Corpulency, when in an extraordinary degree, may be reckoned as a disease, as it in some measure obstructs the free exercise of the animal functions and hath a tendency to shorten life, by paving the way to dangerous distempers.' A number of doctors who came after him jumped on the unhealthy-corpulence bandwagon and began to link an extravagant variety of 'dangerous distempers' to excess weight, many quite spuriously.

Corpulence challenged on aesthetic, health and moral grounds

Corpulence found itself in the dock on three separate charges: it was unattractive, unhealthy and sinful. A comely plumpness might be admired, but extreme corpulence, obesity, as demonstrated by the rotund Prince Regent, was mocked and despised. Doctors started to catalogue health hazards caused or aggravated by overweight. In addition to the obvious joint pain, dyspepsia (indigestion) and breathlessness, it was suggested that gout, carbuncles and even boils could be caused by overweight. Improved understanding of how the body handled different components in food – *proteins*, fats, sugars and starches – inspired British surgeon William Harvey to design the first successful low-*carbohydrate* slimming diet which he prescribed for a patient, William Banting. Banting's spectacular weight loss lent a new word to the dictionary – 'to bant', meaning to diet.

In America, campaigners invoked the sin of gluttony to persuade people to consume less and lose weight. Historian Peter Stearns of George Mason University in the USA argues that the change in attitudes towards obesity during the nineteenth century can be attributed to a guilty reaction to the new abundance of food, the emergence of consumer culture, and the growth of sedentary work habits – something Cheyne had noticed 100 years earlier. Stearns blames the 'religious legacies' of the USA which made dieting the new Puritanism, contrasted with attitudes to weight in France which have remained essentially aesthetic and where dieters have more success than they do in the USA.

Whatever the explanation, diet and health became inextricably bonded to virtue in the American psyche. A minister called Sylvester Graham blamed all manner of immorality on gluttony, and preached that the way to physical, moral and spiritual good health was via a bland, vegetarian diet, again echoing Cheyne. Gluttony led to indigestion, he believed, followed by a state of 'overstimulation' and ultimately illness. He proscribed not only alcohol but tea, coffee and all stimulants. An early advocate of dietary fibre, he recommended coarse-ground whole-wheat flour, from which he created a flat bread called Graham Crackers. (In the USA, what we call digestive biscuits are still referred to as 'Graham Crackers', but they are square.) The culinary appeal of this early health food may be judged by the fact that he became known as 'Dr Sawdust', and although his devotees claimed that the regime promoted health and strength, the unconverted said they looked pale and sickly.

In Victorian times in the UK, health campaigners were preoccupied with the widespread scourge of fatal infections and insanitary living conditions, rather than the risk to the wealthy few of getting too fat. But doctors treating the wealthy were also concerned with the health consequences of overweight. They were aided by technical developments that made it possible to measure blood pressure accurately. This was the forerunner of the modern *sphygmomanometer* – a pressure cuff that temporarily stops the blood flow in the arm so that the sound of the blood rushing back into the blood vessels can be heard with a *stethoscope*, and the pressure exerted by the heart to drive it back measured. It was invented in 1881 by the gloriously named Samuel Siegfried Karl Ritter von Basch. The link between raised blood pressure and fatal heart disease or stroke was already known and now it became clear that blood pressure increased with weight gain.

Measuring overweight

The first people to hit upon the value of calculating 'healthy' weight were, not surprisingly, life insurance salesmen. A connection between overweight and mortality had first been noted by the Greek philosopher–physician Hippocrates in the fifth century BC. 'Sudden death is more common in those who are naturally fat than in the lean,' observed the father of medicine, without attempting an explanation. Physicians like Cheyne and Flemyng had also made the connection between excessive fat and a risk to basic 'animal functions', like breathing and being physically active. By the middle of the nineteenth century, William Banting refers to a healthy weight-for-height ('stature') tabulation drawn up by Dr John Hutchinson for an insurance company and based on the volume of air passing in and out of the lungs. Banting wisely observes that such tabulations only work as averages: '. . . some in health weighing more by many pounds than others. It must not be looked upon as infallible, but only as a sort of general, reasonable, guide to Nature's great and mighty work.'

Hutchinson's calculations did not distinguish between men and women or between different builds; nevertheless, they are considerably more generous than the scales that followed. In 1871, French physician Pierre Paul Broca (famous for identifying the area in the brain where speech is generated and understood) proposed a scale whereby a healthy man's weight (in kilograms) should be the same as the number of centimetres greater than a metre that he measured in height; slightly less in the case of women. This works out as pretty skinny for either sex. Broca derived his 'ideal body weight' idea from the observation that the obese were more likely to have the symptoms of heart disease.

Broca's index probably influenced the tables developed by the insurance industry in the twentieth century. The American Metropolitan Life (Met Life) tables were created in 1943 and charted what was termed 'desirable' height–weight ratios, based on those of people with the lowest mortality rate. They expanded the earlier, simple formulas by proposing different weights for people of the same height but different 'frames'. There was no evidence for the fact that people could be meaningfully divided up into different frames, but the system did at least have the virtue of acknowledging human diversity. On the Met Life scales a woman of average height (5 feet 5 inches) could weigh from 117 pounds (53 kilos) to 155 pounds (70.3 kilos). But 'frame' size was difficult to calculate and approximated only roughly to individual differences in fat, muscle and bone mass, the really important factors contributing to different height–weight ratios. Other limitations to the Met Life scales made them inadequate as a measure of health or a predictor of illness. They calculate height to include a one-inch heel, so we must assume they calculate weight to include clothing. Including a variable of this magnitude makes them even less helpful. Was the guy wearing a three-piece suit and elastic-sided boots or his pyjamas when being weighed? They were supposed to apply to adults aged between 25 and 59. (They are certainly useless if applied to children or adolescents.) But they were, of course, based on life insurance customers, and not that many young people take out life insurance – particularly the case in the 1940s. However, these crude actuarial scales continued to be taken as a guide to what was a healthy weight until, in the 1980s, the body-mass index (BMI) took over.

The rise and rise of the body-mass index

The formula for calculating body mass is: your weight in kilograms divided by your height in metres squared. It's a pain to work out and most people resort to BMI tables. (You can find a table on p. 109.)

Quetelet and 'the average man'

Although BMI only became the preferred way of calculating overweight and obesity in the 1980s, its origins go back even earlier than Hutchinson's insurance tables. It was devised by a Flemish mathematician called Quetelet in the early nineteenth century. Quetelet was keenly interested in the concept of 'the average man', believing that this represented some kind of ideal. (He applied the same mathematical analysis to mortality and to crime.) He plotted the distribution of various physical and mental attributes on a graph that took on the classical 'bell' shape. He identified the maximum central point of the curve as the optimum, or ideal point, and he classified the tail-ends of the curve abnormal and bad. On this basis, he found the average (hence 'ideal') BMI was about 22–23, and declared that people with a BMI over 30 were obese. Now, if you track the mortality of individuals with the same BMI, you find that it also follows a curve, but 'U' shaped, with the lowest point (lowest risk of early death) in the middle, raised at each end. However, this low-risk group are not BMI 22–23, but about 27. This is just one limitation to using BMI as a guide to a healthy weight, and there are others. (See the box on BMI tables on pp. 12–13.)

Some very august bodies have put their weight (so to speak) behind BMI as the gold standard for measuring healthy weight. The interesting thing is that since the 1980s, surveys show people in most countries getting fatter – not just in affluent, developed ones, but also in India, Pakistan and other developing countries. So did the experts revise their recommended 'healthy' weights? No. They did the reverse; as people over the world got fatter, the guidelines for so-called 'healthy' or desirable weight got lower.

To begin with, the guidelines subdivided BMI into underweight, normal, 'marginally overweight', overweight and obese, with two complicated sets of tables for men and women. (See the box on BMI tables on pp. 12–13.) The idea of 'marginal' overweight was new and sensible; the BMI proposed in these tables is still low when compared with average weight of people at the time. But in 2000 the World Health Organization (WHO) and the Centers for Disease Control and Prevention in the USA decided to move the goalposts. Henceforth any adult, male or female, with a BMI of 25 or more was to be considered 'overweight' and at a BMI of 30 he or she was 'obese'. Remember this when you hear that rates of obesity are ballooning out of all proportion: they are not being measured against the same yardstick.

Are we really suffering from an 'obesity epidemic'?

An increasingly vocal number of experts have started to question healthy weight as rated by these mighty health authorities. Some have re-examined the studies most frequently quoted to justify the claim that being overweight or obese makes you ill, and that at the prescribed BMI (25 or less) you are axiomatically healthy – or at any rate health*ier* than at 27, 28 or 29, for example. Two well-argued books and a comprehensive website provide heavyweight backing for the criticisms summarized below (Paul Campos' *The Obesity Myth* and *The Skinny on Fat* by Shawna Vogel, and <www.halls.md.>).

Why crude body-mass index ratings of healthy weight are misleading

- Human beings are not slabs of homogeneous tissue. They are made up of bone, muscle, fat and a variety of organs, all of which have different density and therefore contribute differently to body weight. In general terms, people with large bones or well-developed muscles will be heavier than someone of the same height but lightly boned, even with a generous covering of fat. That is why the Harlem Globetrotters and the All-Blacks have a BMI in the high 20s to 30 or more. It's also why crews in the Oxford and Cambridge Boat Race feature oarsmen who would be considered overweight judged against a BMI of 25, while the cox would be rated underweight. The tall, the large and the well-built are unfairly stigmatized by a rigid rule for healthy weight. By the same score, some races tend to be heavier for the same height than others, and can't be assessed on the same healthy-weight scale. African Americans come out higher, weight for height, and people from Asia, mostly lightly built, lower. All this points to the nonsense of postulating an ideal global BMI of 25.

- Human beings don't have straight sides, nor are they two-dimensional, so it is clearly crazy to calculate their ideal size by dividing their weight by the square of their height. This would only be appropriate for people shaped like road signs. Even if we were to divide their weight by a cubed measurement, it would still be pretty inadequate since they're not built like refrigerators either.

- In addition to professional athletes and some racial groups, BMI is a poor measure of overweight or health risk in children and teenagers because the scales are based on adults' height. And pregnant or breast-feeding women need more fat reserves than at other times. It is even less of a health predictor for people over 65. Even healthy people tend to accumulate body fat and lose bone mass, and ultimately height, as they grow older, leading to changes in BMI unrelated to their health. In fact there is clear evidence that in old age a slightly higher BMI can be protective, providing energy reserves in case of illness.

Measuring fat and its distribution, rather than weight

As Morgagni noted all those years ago, it is the distribution of fat that can cause health problems, rather than body weight per se. Tests that measure the thickness of body fat and its distribution are much better than BMI at calculating whether someone is overweight. A skinfold measure, for example, uses a pair of calipers to measure the thickness of the fat layer on the arm or stomach. This has been used since the early 1900s; it has the advantage that it is measuring actual fat, but the disadvantage that some complicated calculations have to be made to extrapolate for the overall distribution of this tissue.

There is also an electrical device that exploits the fact that muscle has more water in it than fat and therefore is a better conductor of electrical current. Fatty tissues slow down the current, or 'impede' it, so the device is known as *bioelectrical impedance analysis* or BIA. Electrodes are positioned on the wrists or ankles and low-level current passed through the body. Depending on the proportion of fat to muscle, the current will be impeded or pass more easily. Fitting electrodes involves a trained technician at a gym or doctor's surgery, but there are scales that operate on the same basic principle, and even some that make an estimate of the rate at which the body burns up fat, based on the fact that the more muscle you have the higher the rate will be.

Finally, there is the question of fat distribution, as opposed to the overall quantity of body fat. In the 1940s, a French doctor called Jean Vague rediscovered what Morgagni had noted 200 years earlier: that the people most at risk of heart disease, diabetes and gout had fat deposits mainly round their middle – what he called 'centrally' deposited fat, as opposed to 'peripherally', or *android* obesity, because it was more common in men than in women (a 'beer-belly'). This kind of fat deposit, again noticed by Morgagni, is most commonly associated with a build-up of internal fat deposits around the organs – in some cases as much as 60 per cent more than normal. Since then, numerous studies have confirmed the association of this particular fat distribution with a cluster of health problems including insulin resistance (characteristic of type 2 diabetes), high blood pressure, an unhealthy balance of fats in the blood, heart disease and death from these illnesses, which has become known as the *metabolic syndrome.*

Charts were devised to measure the ratio of waist to hip circumference (tricky to calibrate, but the smaller your waist is in relation to your hips, the better), and waist to height ratio (WHTR). Simply put, these last suggest that if your waist measures more than half your height, you may be in trouble health-wise.

About ten years ago a doctor called Margaret Ashwell developed a chart similar to the BMI – the Ashwell Shape Chart – that indicates the health risk as determined by body shape. (You can find it at <http://www.ashwell.uk.com/shape.htm>.) Simply explained, she characterizes fat distribution as 'Apples' or 'Pears'. Apples have excess fat deep down in the region of the stomach, often associated with serious conditions such as heart disease, raised blood pressure, diabetes and some types of cancer. Pears may have excess fat under the skin (subcutaneous fat, the padding that in youth softens the outline of bones), around the bottom, hips and thighs, but this appears to be much less harmful to health.

The attraction of using the Ashwell Shape Chart combined with WHTR is that it appears to be a good predictor of health risk for ethnic groups – like those from Asia and China, who are lightly built with low rates of obesity – and even for children.

When it comes to tracking a relationship with health, I believe that shape and activity level – dealt with in later chapters – turn out to be much more important than weight.

NHANES BMI tables and revised definitions of overweight

(Drawn from the National Health and Nutrition Examination Survey (NHANES) of the dietary habits and health of US residents, conducted every ten years by the National Center for Health Statistics.)

Range	Women	Men
Underweight	Less than 19.1	Less than 20.7
Within normal range	19.1–25.8	20.7–26.4
Marginally overweight	25.8–27.3	26.4–27.8
Overweight	27.3–32.3	27.8–31.1
Very overweight or obese	More than 32.3	More than 31.1

For those of you not yet familiar with working out BMI – you will be –
these translate approximately for the average 5ft 6in (1.62m) woman
as:

Underweight	below 8 st 8 lb (54.5 kilos)
Normal	up to 11 st (70 kilos)
Marginally overweight	up to 11 st 6 lb (72.7 kilos)
Overweight	up to 12 st 1 lb (76.8 kilos)
Obese	up to 14 st 4 lb (90.9 kilos)
Very obese	over 14 st 4 lb

The super-sane Halls.md website, <http://www.halls.md/body-mass-index/age.htm>, provides substantial argument for revising the
recommended BMI upwards based on what it calls 'educated
guessing'.

2

Why do we weigh what we weigh?

If you read anything about health, you will be used to the usual answer to this question: it's a combination of things – nature and nurture; genes and environment; constitution and behaviour. Where weight is concerned, we have been conditioned to think that behaviour is all-important. That infuriatingly thin doctor says smugly, 'Calories in; calories out. It's all a matter of balancing what you eat with the energy you expend. There were no fat people in concentration camps.'

'Well, maybe,' you might answer. Because the fact is, what you weigh is *not* simply a question of balancing what you eat with the energy you expend, although this certainly plays a part. People vary, like cars; their consumption of fuel per miles travelled is not all the same. And that is how they are meant to be. The idea of everyone being the same size and shape – like the line-up in the chorus of the Folies-Bergère – is absurd. Nor are we designed to be the same shape but in different sizes, like Russian dolls. There is certainly no such thing as a 'perfect' weight. There are, of course, physical ideals – the perfect woman or man, as represented by statues of Greek gods or photos of Hollywood film stars – but these, as we discussed in Chapter 1, tend to vary with place and context.

In this book, the concern is not with achieving a perfect or even a healthy weight, in absolute terms. I want to identify, and help you achieve, what is perfect or healthy for *you*. For many, this turns out to be the weight they were when young. This is not universal; some people are podgy or skinny in their teens and only really find their true body weight with maturity. But one thing is virtually universal: the shape and size that is natural to you only emerges at puberty. That is when a tendency to have a big bottom, powerful shoulders or full breasts becomes apparent.

Children are generally less physically distinctive than adults. Baby-fat apart, fat children, and to a lesser extent very thin children, are usually unhealthy or unhappy. However, if at 18 Joe discovers he has the build to play rugby and Jenny develops the curves of a Rubens Venus, it does not imply that they are less healthy than Jane and John, contemporaries who develop the figures to take up modelling.

Worries about weight usually come later in life. Not all, I know – the teens can be a time of intense worry about body image, particularly for girls. But what I am trying to establish is that, even when people are in the prime of life, they are not all the same, and, just as their heights vary, so will their body mass in relation to their height. *Vive la différence!* Variety is the spice of life. Which factors make us so varied?

It all starts in the genes

Did your mother stay slim, despite having children? Was your father athletic? Do you come from a line of sturdy, farming stock, bred for labouring in the fields? Physical build is something that we clearly inherit from our forebears. But the exact blend is shaken up in the cocktail mixer of sexual reproduction. Your parents actually carry hidden genes for physical characteristics that they do not exhibit because in their particular genetic cocktail the gene is *recessive*: that is, it is suppressed by a matching dominant gene that overrides it. But once that parent's recessive gene passes down to the next generation, it may find itself paired with a gene from the other parent that is also recessive, so that the characteristic it confers – musical talent or heavy thighs – will suddenly reappear, having missed out a generation.

The debate about nature and nurture goes to and fro like the tide among scientists. The science of why we put on weight (let's be bold and use the dreaded word 'obesity' science) is no exception. The idea that being overweight or obese is sinful, considered in Chapter 1, has its roots in the nurture explanation: people get fat because they have grown up eating too much, or the wrong things. But in recent years the nature explanation has received a massive boost with increased understanding of how the genes we inherit affect not only how our bodies are constructed – how much muscle, how large the bones, how much fat – but how our bodies convert food into energy (metabolize it) and how various *neurotransmitters*, the chemical messengers in the brain, affect our appetite, mood and general behaviour.

The nurture–nature debate is confounded by the fact that the vast majority of us are nurtured by the parents from whom we inherited our nature or genes, so it can be difficult to tell whether it is a mother's genes or her fantastic way with pastry that have made her children as roly-poly as she is!

Julie's story

When I first met Julie, she was a highly successful businesswoman in her late twenties. She was bright, articulate, attractive and funny, but always seemed rather shy with men. I remember noticing as slightly odd that Julie always wore long skirts – in the age of the mini-skirt. I put it down to her shyness. But when I got to know her better I learned that the real reason was that she had disproportionately massive thighs (I can say this freely having used a pseudonym for Julie as I do for all the case histories in this book). Julie had a fantastic swimming pool, but I never saw her swim when people were there. She ate like a bird, and as I got to know her better I learned that she was worried that her strenuous dieting would make her flat-chested. We lost touch but some years later I received a wedding invitation. I was unable to attend but hoped that true love would have made Julie accept her body as it was, thighs and all. Imagine my distress when the next I heard of her was an obituary in *The Times.* I phoned a mutual friend and learned the sad story. Desperate to lose what she saw as those awful thighs before getting married, Julie had gone on a starvation diet and also undergone *liposuction* (a cosmetic procedure to remove superficial fat with a suction pump). In the weakened state that comes with excessive dieting she had caught an infection which had developed into pneumonia, and in hospital had contracted septicaemia and died. It was the most tragic case I have ever come across of rejecting the body to which you were born. Julie's thighs were no bigger than those of the Willendorf Venus. She was an attractive, successful young woman. She killed herself trying to thwart her genes.

This dramatic anecdote illustrates the degree to which shape and size are in our genes. People can modify body shape to some degree with body-building exercise or plastic surgery, as well as, more prosaically, by consuming too many calories, but the underlying blueprint is laid down immutably in their DNA. Life experience may modify the expression of our body-shaping genes: illness or privation in childhood may stunt growth just as an unhealthy lifestyle of too much junk food may incline you to put on weight, but these environmental pressures will affect individuals differently depending on the inclination to be tall or short, muscular or weedy, plump or skinny that is written in their DNA.

Enter the obese mouse

Much research on weight and health is in the form of *epidemiological studies* – the branch of science that studies health or disease by recording what happens in whole populations. But to understand what actually goes on in the individual body or brain that makes one person heavier than another, or makes one put on weight while the other stays slim, requires more intrusive techniques. Doing research on human beings is quite rightly hedged around with ethical restrictions, and breakthroughs in science often start with discoveries about what happens in experimental animals, usually mice or rats.

The first obesity gene, the OB gene, was reported in 1994 by scientists at the Rockefeller University in New York, who identified the variant of gene that made a breed of laboratory mice fat. They discovered a hormone which they called *leptin* – from the Greek word for 'thin' – that regulates body weight. It is produced predominantly in the fat cells in the body, but also in the lining of the stomach, and appears to be part of the mechanism by which the body knows whether to store fat or burn it off. Leptin communicates with the area in the brain that controls the rate at which the body burns up energy (the metabolic rate), turning it up or down depending on whether the mouse needs nourishment or has eaten enough. The OB mice lacked leptin-receptors, so messages to stop eating because they were full didn't get through, and they just kept stuffing themselves. Leptin given to normal mice made them lose weight.

When in 2003 the *Human Genome Project* published the outline blueprint of human genes, researchers discovered that the same variant of the OB gene in mice also occurred in obese humans. Was leptin the magic bullet for dieters? Would a daily dose of leptin do for overweight humans what it did for normal mice? Leptin replacement did work for some rather rare forms of obesity in children, but it didn't work for everyone who was overweight. The discovery was more important for disposing of the idea that people were totally responsible for what they weighed. It did not, at a stroke, imply that human beings could blame their beer-bellies on their genes. Most genes make you *inclined* towards some trait or other. They do not dictate an immutable outcome. Nevertheless, it was a landmark in that it provided an explanation for why some people put on weight other than simply 'Calories in and calories out'. As Shawna Vogel puts it in her book *The Skinny on Fat*:

> Virtually overnight, it introduced millions of people to the idea that overweight was not a personality defect. You don't have to be a sloth or a glutton to be fat. The obese (mouse) discovery substantiated what many had long suspected – that weight problems lurk in some people's DNA.

And obese children

Several other genes that confer a tendency to put on weight have also been discovered. Because the tendency is inherited, the effects tend to show up in children. Another gene affects the production of the hormone *insulin*. It is the body's failure to produce insulin, or to respond to it, which causes diabetes, and insulin is known to play a key role in the processing of fat in the body as well as the breakdown of sugars.

Another gene controls not only appetite regulation but the body's manufacture of the pigments that colour skin and hair (such children are red-haired and freckly). Professor Steve O'Rahilly, head of the Department of Clinical Biochemistry and Medicine at the University of Cambridge, has to date identified seven different obesity genes present in obese children or their families.

Although these variants explain many cases of childhood obesity, they go only a small way to explain the more complex variations in weight and weight gain in adults, and most are either rare or found in many people who are not obese, as well as some who are. While I was writing this book, a team at Boston University in the USA, led by Michael Christman, announced that they had located the first relatively common genetic variant that increased the risk of obesity.

This gene controls insulin – in fact, it is induced by insulin and interferes with the *synthesis* (manufacturing in the body) of fatty acid and cholesterol (the building blocks of fat). Because they are unable to inhibit the synthesis of fatty acid and cholesterol, people with a particular variant of this gene tend to accumulate fat and put on weight more easily. The variant appears to be present in some 10 per cent of the population, and it increases their risk of getting overweight by as much as 50 per cent. 'The predisposition to obesity that it causes is modest, but it's present in so many people that it represents a major cause of obesity,' said Christman in the journal *Science*.

Weight and body mass remain a multi-factorial phenomenon. These discoveries advance our understanding of the mechanism of weight control, but have not greatly advanced the treatment of obesity. Leptin replacement for children with a faulty leptin-producing gene is a rare example of a gene discovery leading directly to a therapeutic intervention. Nevertheless, the goal enabling people to eat what they like and stay slim shimmers like a vision of the Holy Grail over drug research and in the mind of everyone who has ever tried to diet.

What are obesity genes for?

Why do such genes occur? As we will see in Chapter 3, severely obese people are susceptible to several serious medical conditions, in particular type 2 diabetes. It shortens life and reduces fertility. True, it is more likely to occur as people get older – after they have had a family and passed on their obesity genes – but nevertheless it is a conundrum that bothers scientists. What they suggest is that genes that make people able to put on weight easily could have been very useful at times or in countries where food shortages were a constant hazard.

The idea, known as the 'thrifty gene hypothesis', was first proposed by James Neel of the University of Michigan medical school in the 1960s, and subsequently many more researchers have elaborated on it. It is supported by the fact that obesity genes and the incidence of type 2 diabetes are more prevalent in several distinct populations: American Indians, Australian Aborigines and Pacific Islanders. Genes that predispose people to gain weight in times of plenty would have had a selective advantage in populations that often experienced starvation or frequent food shortages, such as occurred during the initial colonization of 'new worlds', according to anthropologist M. Wendorf from the University of California, Berkeley: 'The "thrifty" genotype (obesity genes) may have once allowed founding populations to survive feast or famine conditions for several generations. With an assured food supply and a sedentary lifestyle, however, the "thrifty" genotype becomes disadvantageous.'

Experience in the womb

Let's consider an influence which, although not genetic – it is nurture in the purest sense – is nevertheless nothing to do with what you do, and is way beyond your control. A team under Professor David Barker at the University of Southampton has observed that it is the rate of weight gain in childhood, not the degree of fatness at any one time, which is the main predictor of future health problems. The team studied the medical records of 8,760 Finnish people. The results showed that children who were small and thin up to the age of two and gained weight more quickly than their peers thereafter, catching up with, or even surpassing them, by the age of 11, were most at risk of health problems as adults. Those who demonstrated this pattern of growth as children grew up to be resistant to the effects of insulin (type 2 diabetes) and were most likely to develop the risk factors that predisposed them to heart disease.

Conversely, infants who grew rapidly in the first two years of life, whatever their ultimate size, were less likely to experience *coronary heart disease* as adults. 'Under-nutrition in the womb and slow early development may programme a "thrifty" metabolism, which includes insulin resistance, and which becomes inappropriate with adequate or excess nutrition in childhood,' said Professor Barker. (More about Barker's hypothesis in Chapter 5.)

We have discussed the natural variations in build and the contribution of genes, and so arrive at the environmental and behavioural factors that affect weight.

Starve now; die later

There is one curious exception to the principle that starvation – the preferred term is 'calorie restriction' (CR) – makes you ill. It has been known for many years that CR enables laboratory mice to stay healthy, prolong function and increase their lifespan by 40 per cent, and several primate studies are under way. George Roth and his team at the US National Institute on Aging in Baltimore, USA, enrolled his first Rhesus monkey for a 30 per cent CR trial more than 17 years ago, and the latest bulletin from his ongoing research programme confirms that these monkeys are indeed healthier, have about half the death rate, and maintain a lot of different physical functions, better than monkeys that are allowed to eat all they want. Since the maximum lifespan for this primate in captivity is about 40 years, Roth has some way to go before he can quantify an increase in simian lifespan.

So far no one has been able to induce human beings to enter into a controlled trial of 30 per cent CR, although a team at the Washington University School of Medicine studied a small group of 25 middle-aged men who had voluntarily restricted their calories to between 1,000 and 2,000 a day for six years, and found that they had greatly reduced all the risk factors for heart disease and diabetes. Members of the US Caloric Restriction Optimal Nutrition Society (<www.calorierestriction.org>) try to consume between 10 and 25 per cent fewer calories than average Americans while still maintaining proper nutrition. They emphasize that CR is not about starvation, but eliminating calories by eating nutrient-dense foods.

'Food, glorious food'

In the modern welfare state few of us go short of food. In the developing world the rains may fail or the locusts eat your harvest. A lion must hunt to make a kill, a fox overturn a rubbish bin to make sure of supper, but for us food is always available, at the clunk of a fridge door, the plonk of a vending machine or the tinkle of a cash register. We don't eat because we're hungry and need to survive, but for a plethora of other reasons: because it is mealtime; because we see food and are tempted; because everyone else is eating; because we are bored, anxious or depressed. It is the first human satisfaction we experience (nipple, teat or thumb) and we often resort to it when in need of comfort, or when we have nothing better to do.

In the wild, no animal is overweight. In the laboratory, with food supplied on demand, animals can become as fat as some humans. For us, eating has become remote from consuming fuel to supply our energy needs. What with cars, lifts and remote-controls, our energy needs have shrunk, so many of us consume more than our bodies can dispose of in energy. If the mixture is too rich in a petrol engine, spare fuel escapes in the exhaust. If human beings have too rich a mixture, their bodies may store it – as fat.

The most direct way in which food contributes to weight is obviously related to how much of it you eat. It's not a direct relationship – eat a pound of steak and weigh a pound more on the scales – because to convert steak into you (to metabolize it) requires that your body burn up energy to break it down into an absorbable form, and some of it, that can't be absorbed, will end up as waste.

While the overall quantity of food you consume is the principal way food contributes to weight, the kind of food also counts, especially if you are still growing, growing a baby, or using up masses of energy as a navvy or a ballet dancer. In all these cases you will need more protein – the basic building blocks of tissue. Which particular foods you eat will also contribute to the rate at which you burn it up in calories. Fans of the Atkins diet claim that if you eat a lot of protein but no carbohydrate – sugars, starches and such – you will put up the rate you burn off calories by more than your intake, and this will mean your body has to draw upon fat reserves and you lose weight.

Another way that the kind of food you eat affects what you weigh is in how it affects your appetite. Fat takes longer for the body to break down, so that it will generally take longer for you to feel hunger after a hunk of cheese than after the equivalent amount of rice or bread. But here we come to a problem. Not everyone burns off the calories they eat at the same rate.

Understanding energy consumption

Let us return to 'Calories in; calories out'. People trying to lose weight tend to concentrate on the former, but the latter is every bit as important. And, as with everything affecting the shape and size of your body, burning up calories is not as straightforward as it is sometimes made out to be. Once again, behaviour – how much energy you expend running up and down stairs, digging the garden or lifting weights – is only part of the story. Different bodies burn up calories at a different rate, and the same body burns them up at a different rate depending on the circumstances.

What we are talking about here is the metabolic rate: the rate at which food, or stored food in the form of fat, is converted into energy. Unfortunately, people are not like cars: you can't estimate their consumption by the amount of fuel you have to put in to travel 100 miles. Most calculations of metabolic rate are incredibly crude: as crude, in fact, as the estimates of what a person of a given height should weigh. It is possible to calculate what an individual's metabolic rate is when at rest – the resting metabolic rate (RMR) – or to calculate what he or she burns over a 24-hour period which will include sleep, rest, light and some vigorous activity, but the equipment to do this is complicated and expensive. A simpler system measures the oxygen people use while at rest, which has a direct relation to the calories they burn.

Most people appreciate that exercise puts up the metabolic rate but, activity apart, many factors – environmental as well as individual – affect its base level.

- Body composition – lean or muscular people have a higher RMR; those with more fat have a lower one.
- Height – tall, thin people have a higher RMR.
- Age – the younger you are, the higher your RMR. It slows down with age.
- Growth – growing children and pregnant women have a higher RMR.
- Environmental temperature – heat and cold raise RMR; the body uses energy maintaining body temperature.
- Fever – body temperature goes up, so does the RMR.
- Stress – the hormones produced to cope with stress may raise RMR.
- Malnutrition – lowers RMR.
- Starvation or fasting – the body produces hormones that lower RMR.

- Thyroxin – this hormone, produced in the *thyroid gland*, is central to the regulation of the metabolic rate; deficiencies in production lower RMR, over-production raises it.

(Based on the Cornell University Nutritional Sciences 421 Sports Nutrition webpage, <http://instruct1.cit.cornell.edu/Courses/ns421/BMR.html>)

Low and lower, and high and higher RMR

The Pima Indians from Arizona in the southern United States and Mexico are a much studied group because, although they have significant genes and physiology in common, those who live in the USA have a pronounced tendency to put on weight and develop type 2 diabetes while those in Mexico do not. In the 1990s Eric Ravussin, a scientist at the National Institute of Diabetes and Digestive and Kidney Diseases in Phoenix, Arizona, uncovered some interesting variations among Pima Indians who in general exhibit a low RMR. He found that there was a threefold difference in the amount of food his research subjects could burn up in a given 24-hour period: 3,015 compared with 1,067. This was not a measure of RMR, but of an average day's energy consumption. Taking account of the physical and environmental factors affecting metabolic rate (he also included gender differences, which make women likely to have lower metabolic rates than men, weight for weight) he still found a large range of metabolic rates within this low metabolic rate population.

Unfortunately, this doesn't mean that everyone carrying too much weight has a lower than average RMR – would that it were so simple. Nevertheless, Ravussin did find that a person's RMR was a good predictor of whether they would gain weight over a four-year period. However, the researchers found that only 40 per cent of the weight gain could be accounted for by the differences in metabolism. The rest was contributed by food consumption (calories in) and daily energy expenditure in activity (calories out).

Research on athletes indicates another interesting variation in RMR. It is not something fixed; behaviour modifies it. A study of a small group of male athletes in the prime of life was carried out at Hyderabad, India, by scientists at the Institute of Nutrition. They were interested in the nutritional requirements of a professional athlete in training for competition, so they measured the basal metabolic rate (the resting rate with the rate when sleeping added in – in other words, the very lowest metabolic rate) while the athletes were in training, pre-competition and during competition: and, as you may have guessed, their metabolic rates increased. The athletes also increased their lean body mass and a number of other measures of overall fitness, and the study concluded that metabolic rate was directly related to the level of training being undertaken at the time.

These measures of fitness – pulse rate (and the time it takes to return to normal after exercise), heart rate, respiration rate, maximum intake of oxygen (known as *VO2max*) – are all thought to be related to the basal metabolic rate, and the beneficial role of regular exercise is usually measured against them. But even here individuals vary. Canadian researcher Claude Bouchard has done a number of studies on how people responded to exercise, and – yes, you've guessed – there turns out to be a fivefold difference in the way their bodies respond (in this case) to two hours a day on an exercise bike for a total of 22 days. Bouchard's non-responders were young men in the prime of life, like the Indian athletes, so their failure to respond cannot be attributed to ageing. All the indicators are that, just as there are people who gain weight on relatively low calorie consumption, there are also those who don't have the option of burning off calories by pedalling away at the exercise! Isn't life unfair?

But all is not lost. In Chapter 8 we will return to the value of exercise in maintaining a healthy weight. In the meantime there is reassurance from the American College of Sports Medicine: people who do at least moderate amounts of activity feel a great deal better than those who do not.

I fear that this is a rather unsatisfactory ending for this chapter. We have seen that the factors that contribute to what each of us weighs are infinitely complex. Almost certainly some are beyond our control – our genes, how our bodies are constructed and whether they make it easy for us to put on weight and difficult to take it off. Ultimately, however, it is worth remembering that being a certain weight is not a meaningful goal in its own right. It is being healthy and happy that matters. If you are these, the chances are that the weight you are is right for you.

3

Are there health risks related to weight?

Time to face it straight on: can weight be a health risk?

And of course the answer is, 'It depends.' It depends on what you personally weigh in relation to your height; where you fall on all these various charts – the body-mass index (BMI), the Met Life mortality scales, the Ashwell charts of body shape – and above all what your general health is like. But the answer also depends on something else. It depends on which expert you choose to ask, because they simply do not agree. Calculating what illnesses people are likely to get based purely on what they weigh or how fat they are (or BMI, or body shape or skinfold) is frankly a mug's game. The studies that are cited as the scientific basis of the hysterical claim that we have 'an epidemic of obesity' in the UK, USA or the rest of the world, or that we are all going to fall off our perches at an early age because we are greedy couch-potatoes, are in no way as clear-cut as the studies that show that if you are a smoker you have a very high chance of developing lung cancer or coronary artery disease and ultimately dying of it. They can be interpreted differently, and they are. The health risks related to being overweight or obese have not been plotted on some perfectly calibrated medical scale that would enable you to slide your finger up until you found your BMI, follow it along the line and discover '50 per cent chance of getting breast cancer by the age of 60', '30 per cent chance of having raised blood pressure by 65' or '20 per cent chance of developing type 2 diabetes by the time you are 50'.

If you approach the relationship between overweight and illness the other way round, it is a little easier to say something meaningful. However, most of the information on the relationship between health and weight comes from studies of populations. They provide only a very approximate idea of individual risk. In general, one can say that the medical conditions listed on p. 30 appear to be slightly more prevalent among groups of people carrying 'extra' weight than among those of so-called 'normal' weight, but this is not a measure of individual risk and it is quite small – sometimes as low as perhaps two people in every 10,000. To have any bearing on the health of individuals, population studies need to demonstrate a really massive difference between one group and another – as they do for the risk of lung cancer among smokers compared with non-smokers: nine to ten times higher.

As we have seen, the experts don't even agree on what 'normal' weight is. Quetelet, who devised the BMI, settled on 25 because it fell at the mid-line of a graph showing the distribution of adult BMI (see the box on Quetelet and 'the average man', p. 8). Nowadays the mean BMI in most populations falls nearer 26–27, a level common among well-built or athletic people which is no hindrance to physical activity. The WHO settled on a BMI of 25 because on graphs plotting risk of death (mortality) against BMI, those at most risk are always at either extreme (under- as well as overweight), and 25 is in the middle of the distribution curve. But so are BMI 27–29 in some populations.

Fatal fat – '300,000 extra deaths'?

If you put '300,000 deaths attributable to obesity' into the Internet search engine Google you get more than 47,000 hits. I didn't read them all, but in the one at the top Paul Campos, a law professor at the University of Colorado in the USA and author of the book *The Obesity Myth* discusses the use of this figure widely promulgated by the US Centers for Disease Control and Prevention (CDC), and explodes it.

The CDC claim that obesity was the cause of an estimated 300,000 preventable deaths per year in the USA, second only to smoking as a fatal 'risk behaviour', originally appeared in the *Journal of the American Medical Association* (*JAMA*) in 1999. Campos calls this paper 'junk science'. According to Glenn Gaesser, a professor of exercise physiology at the University of Virginia, himself author of *Big Fat Lies*, the CDC consulted a number of population studies and found an association between increased weight and slightly higher than average death rate, and attributed this to the extra weight. However, says Gaesser,

The authors made no attempt to determine whether other factors – such as physical inactivity, low fitness levels, poor diet, risky weight-loss practices, and less than adequate access to health care, just to name a few – could have explained some, or all, of the excess mortality in fat people.

Campos adds that the *JAMA* paper also neglected to consider factors such as class and wealth – the poor have worse health than the rich and more of them die early. In short, he says, 'The claim that fat causes 300,000 deaths per year should be dismissed as an assertion for which there is essentially no evidence.'

And bingo, do you know what? A few years later, in November 2004, the CDC were compelled to admit that their figures for preventable deaths that they had attributed to the 'risk behaviour' of being obese were wrong. The deaths were in fact attributable to 'poor diet and physical inactivity'. Gaesser and Campos one; CDC nil.

So far, so good, for the active, well-nourished, possibly overweight. Evidence supporting stronger influences upon health and longevity than weight per se comes from the Cooper Institute in Dallas, USA. The Institute tracked tens of thousands of people for more than ten years and concluded that any excess mortality associated with increased weight could be accounted for by reduced levels of physical activity. Findings like this emerge again and again in the re-evaluation of health–weight studies: moderately active, heavy people (moderate activity being measured in terms of a brisk 30-minute walk each day) have lower mortality rates than thin, inactive people, and effectively the same mortality rates as thin, active people. In other words, factor in the activity variable, and excess weight is no longer a cause of preventable death.

So, the principal studies used to support the contention of 'deaths attributable to obesity' appear to have a case against only the most severely obese, and the point at which increased risk clocks in has also been revised. Data from the National Health and Nutrition Examination Surveys, published in the *Journal of the American Medical Association* in April 2005, show that the level at which overweight was rated (26–29 BMI) is actually optimal in terms of longevity.

But let us look at something else. These studies refer only to preventable deaths among those under 65. As a percentage of total deaths, these are very low, partly because they are for 'preventable' deaths which rules out all killer diseases, such as heart disease, cancer and stroke, but also because the vast majority of deaths in developed countries occur *after* 65 – 78 per cent in the USA and 82 per cent in the UK – so what we are being shown are *very small increases* in the death rate of a *very small percentage* of the population, only among the excessively overweight. After 65, preventable deaths constitute an even smaller percentage of the total and then, most sources agree, *over*weight ceases to become even a minor factor. It is being *under*weight that puts you at increased risk of death once you are over 65.

Figures that don't add up

If you have a feeling for figures you may have been a bit worried about CDC's 300,000 preventable annual US deaths attributed originally to obesity and later to poor diet and inactivity. Approximately 2.3 million Americans die each year; the majority (78 per cent) are over 65. That leaves only 22 per cent of deaths in the under-65 age-group, or about 506,000 annual deaths. This total would include not only those attributed to 'poor diet and inactivity' but also those attributed to all other 'preventable' causes – from smoking to suicide, and road accidents to microbial infection – and also of course the *un*preventable causes of death – cancer, heart attack and stroke. To quote Glenn Gaesser again: 'To suggest that 60 per cent (i.e. three hundred thousand) of these deaths are due to body fat is absolutely preposterous.'

To sum up: extremes of overweight and underweight may make a small contribution to increased risk of death in the young; past the 65th birthday, only underweight increases risk, and even on this some say the jury is still out. The WHO defines obesity as 'a condition of abnormal or excessive fat accumulation in adipose tissue, to the extent that *health may be impaired*'. The extent to which obesity 'impairs health' is estimated by comparing excess fat or high BMI with the occurrence of the various medical conditions in the next section, and even then the evidence is not undisputed. At all events, this definition would seem to class obesity as a *symptom of ill health* rather than a *cause of death*.

Can being too heavy make me ill?

The conditions associated with being overweight are:

- joint disorders (*arthritis* – inflammation of the joints);
- digestive problems like heartburn and *hiatus hernia*;
- breathing difficulties including asthma, chronic bronchitis and obstructive sleep apnoea (OSA) – when someone stops breathing during sleep, usually during snoring, which can be a cause of extreme fatigue or even death;
- breast and other cancers;
- *cardiovascular* disease (relating to the heart and blood vessels, therefore heart disease and stroke) – this is associated with other risk factors: raised blood pressure, high cholesterol and other fats in the blood, hardening and narrowing of the arteries;
- type 2 diabetes, where the body becomes resistant to insulin and cannot break down the carbohydrates and sugars in food.

You can see that some of these, like joint problems, breathing problems and even some digestive problems, are intuitively persuasive because we can see that carrying around extra pounds might aggravate the wear and tear on joints, and that excess adipose tissue (fat) around the abdomen – around the internal organs as well as under the belt – could put pressure on the digestive or breathing organs. Nevertheless, intuition is not evidence, so let's see if science backs it up.

Joint disorders (arthritis)

Many studies support the claim that being overweight increases the risk of developing *osteoarthritis* (OA) – the degenerative form of arthritis caused mostly by wear and tear – in the knee. The exact mechanism by which this occurs is poorly understood. Extra pounds clearly increase the load on joints like the knee, hip or ankle, and increased stress could hasten the breakdown of cartilage, the lining of the joints, that characterizes this form of arthritis. However, overweight is also associated with higher rates of OA in the hands – not normally load-bearing joints – suggesting that some other body system, such as the circulation, may be involved (see 'Cardiovascular disease' on p. 34). Also, many people who are not overweight, including those who damage their joints during sporting activity in youth, get this common condition in middle to old age.

How much extra risk and how much extra weight? Here we return to the familiar problem. Nearly all the studies that link overweight with various health risks are population-based. These give us an idea of trends, but are not very useful for predicting an individual's health risk. Second, characterizing overweight or obesity by the crude yardstick of BMI makes no provision for individual build.

But even viewed with these reservations, the data quoted by the website of the leading US hospital and medical research centre, Johns Hopkins University, in Baltimore, makes a strong case: overweight women have nearly four times the risk of developing knee OA than those of normal weight, and among overweight men it is five times greater. Weight put on in their thirties makes people more likely to develop OA later in life, and losing weight reduces the symptoms – pain, stiffness and reduced mobility – of OA. For the health problems associated with losing weight, see Chapter 4.

It is worth noting that another condition of ageing bones – *osteoporosis* (loss of bone density leading to fragile, breaking bones) – is inversely related to weight. That is, the underweight are more at risk than the overweight. Osteoporosis is a problem for many post-menopausal women, and in the UK more women die following the complications of osteoporosis-related hip fracture than from the gender-related cancers of the breast, womb and cervix combined. (See 'Cancer' on pp. 33–4.)

Digestive problems

The idea is widely held that there is an association between overweight or obesity and symptoms of the variously named indigestion, heartburn, hiatus hernia or *gastro-oesophageal reflux disease* (GORD), to give it its full medical name. However, early studies have been contradictory, although the incidences of both overweight and GORD are increasing in parallel. In GORD (GERD in the USA) corrosive digestive juices from the stomach force their way back through the valve at the top of the stomach, sometimes arriving in the mouth, and damage the lining of the oesophagus, causing pain, ulceration and, in extreme cases, cancer. In 2003 a randomized controlled trial of eradication of *Helicobacter pylori* (a sneaky little bacterium that hides in the gut wall and causes ulcers and other digestive problems) was carried out by the Bristol Helicobacter Project, looking at a large number of patients aged 20–59 years. (This was not a population study, although it appeared in the *International Journal of Epidemiology*.) It measured reflux in terms of frequency and severity of the patient's symptoms and established a clear relationship between GORD and increased BMI. The researchers found that being above normal weight substantially increases the likelihood of suffering heartburn and acid regurgitation, and that someone who is obese is almost three times more likely to experience symptoms than someone of normal weight.

Breathing problems

Here we have a more complex picture. Some conditions such as chronic obstructive pulmonary disease (COPD), also known as emphysema, a progressive lung disease characterized by difficulty in breathing, wheezing and a chronic cough, are more frequently associated with *under*weight. However, several studies in the UK, Sweden and the USA have found that people who develop chronic bronchitis or asthma – a wheezing condition, where the lining of the respiratory tract becomes inflamed and narrowed, usually as some form of allergic reaction – are more likely to be obese. This holds true for both sexes and for children. One study found that men with a waist measurement of over a metre (42 inches) – the Ashwell 'apple' body shape – were most at risk.

A number of factors have been cited to explain why increased weight, especially around the abdomen, should increase the risk of asthma. According to a study at the Harvard School of Public Health, obese people often have lungs that are under-expanded and take smaller breaths, which makes it more likely that their airways will narrow. It found that there was also chronic low-grade systemic inflammation in the obese that appeared to originate in fat tissue and might be causing the airways to narrow excessively. Finally, it discovered that levels of the hormone leptin were higher in the obese than in the lean. Leptin is known to encourage inflammation and higher levels are found among asthmatics even when they are not overweight. However, Jeffrey Fredberg, a co-author of the study, commented, 'Obesity has the capacity to impact lung function in a variety of ways. None of them are good and all of them are poorly understood.'

Another breathing problem more likely to affect the overweight, the obese and especially men, is obstructive sleep apnoea (OSA). *Apnoea* is the Greek for 'no breath', and in OSA people actually stop breathing for ten seconds or more during sleep, maybe as much as several times an hour. It is thought that as many as 1 per cent of the population suffers from the condition, which is also associated with snoring and with having a particular set to the jaw that makes it fall open more easily during sleep. Quite how extra weight is implicated is not totally clear, but fat around the neck appears to be principally to blame, because the tendency to have OSA correlates better with neck circumference than with general obesity. A neck circumference of more than 43 cm (17 inches) is the most significant predictor of problems, and it is thought that the sheer mass of tissue may exert pressure on the windpipe and make it impossible to maintain a clear airway once conscious muscle-tone is relaxed during sleep. Even if the interruption of breathing is not fatal, it can leave the sufferer feeling tired and irritable during the day with a tendency to drop off, in itself dangerous. OSA may also contribute to raised blood pressure and an irregular heart beat – health risks in their own right (see pp. 34, 35 and 36).

Cancer

Oh dear, the picture is no clearer here. Put 'overweight and breast cancer' into a Google search on the Internet and you are deluged with the claim that being overweight as a young adult puts a woman at greater risk from breast cancer after the menopause. But look again: most of the studies are of populations, not controlled trials measuring differences between groups of individuals. If an 'overweight' woman is said to have a 13 per cent increased risk of dying of post-menopausal breast cancer compared to 'normal' weight women, it sounds at first quite alarming. But the devil is in the detail. It is 13 per cent of the not very great risk of any post-menopausal woman dying of breast cancer. Expressed another way, it means that in every 10,000 overweight women, approximately *one* more will die from breast cancer than among 10,000 normal weight women. Epidemiologists usually ignore such small differences because they could so easily be caused by some totally unrelated variable that wasn't factored into the study.

In *Big Fat Lies*, Glenn Gaesser counted some 35 and 40 studies on overweight and cancer over the past 30 years that found an association between increasing body mass and a *lower* incidence of cancer and lower mortality from cancer. The classic Seven Countries Study comparing diet, lifestyle and various risk factors affecting disease in contrasted national populations in the 1960s and 1970s says, 'Relative body weight was an important negative risk factor, meaning that the risk of dying from cancer decreased with increasing relative weight.'

Cardiovascular disease

I saved the last two conditions on the list – cardiovascular disease and type 2 diabetes – until the end because they are the most heavily promoted associations with overweight and the most serious. The mantra is everywhere: being overweight increases your risk of developing circulation problems, heart disease and stroke – the three principal components of cardiovascular disease. Let us look closely at the evidence.

Heart disease and stroke are major causes of death in developed countries like the UK, the USA and Australia. The numbers of people said to be overweight and obese in these countries are also said to be increasing. But hold on a minute: the death rate for heart disease and stroke is actually *coming down* while this alleged *rise* in obesity is taking place. It is less than half what it was a generation ago – the time when the 'obesity epidemic' is said to have begun. So what is happening? Are we getting the diseases but staying alive? A generation ago we were always reading of men in their fifties dropping dead of a heart attack or stroke. Not so today.

Caroline's story
Caroline's father and grandfather both died of sudden heart attacks in their sixties. She doesn't know whether there were warning signs – apart, that is, from her father noting what his own father died of. They

were not thin, but then neither were they noticeably fat. However, when Caroline was undergoing ante-natal care, alarm bells rang because her blood pressure rose, she got puffy ankles (*oedema*) and there were traces of protein in her urine (*proteinuria*) – both signs that her kidneys were not coping. This combination of symptoms, known as *pre-eclampsia*, if not controlled could lead to convulsions, coma and even maternal death, as in the past. Caroline, being a child of a more health-aware age, did take note of the family link with heart disease. She never smoked, she took regular exercise and watched her diet, weight and blood pressure.

Sure enough, in her sixties this last began to creep up. Caroline's health-pride was injured. She became even more strenuous with exercise and diet, and for a while held the rise at bay. Her GP reassured her: it was not lack of discipline on her part that caused the rise, but almost certainly something in her genes. But this was in the 1990s. There were drugs to control high blood pressure that were not widely used when Caroline's father had been her age and were unknown in her grandfather's time. Caroline takes her pills and has moved into a healthy eighth decade. 'If only my father had been living in the same period as me, he might have lived much longer,' says Caroline, somewhat illogically.

The WHO justifies calling obesity a disease because it is associated with an increased incidence of various unhealthy conditions compared with those of normal weight. But, as Michael Gard and Jan Wright document in great detail in *The Obesity Epidemic: Science, Morality and Ideology*, the relative incidence of illness in populations is only a very rough indication of individual risk, unless the difference is massive – as is the risk of death from lung cancer among smokers and non-smokers – and where cardiovascular disease is concerned the additional risk to those of a BMI of more than 30, for example, is quite small. They illustrate this relative risk with reference to the mortality rate for heart disease among New Zealand men. Let us suppose that the risk among obese men were twice the average, then, since 14 per cent of men are obese you would expect twice that number (28 per cent) to die of the disease each year (312 per 100,000) – or 87 out of every 312. That would still leave a massive 72 per cent of non-obese men dying of the disease; nearly three times the rate for the obese men!

I am reminded of the drinker told that 20 per cent of traffic accidents involve a driver over the drink-drive limit. 'Eighty per cent of accidents caused by sober drivers!' he exclaims. 'We've got to get them off the road.'

Most people (most doctors, actually) take it as a given that the risk of developing *coronary artery or heart disease* increases in relation to increased body weight. The connection is persuasive: fats are carried around the body in the blood; some of them get deposited in the walls of the vessels, reducing elasticity, narrowing them and obstructing the flow, particularly that of the vital arteries delivering nutrient-rich blood to the heart (the coronary arteries), to the point where the muscle walls of the heart may be damaged by fuel-starvation, known as *ischaemia* or *infarction*. The narrowing of the blood vessels may increase the pressure the heart has to exert in order to pump the blood round the body (raised blood pressure), at the same time putting it under a strain it may be unable to meet (heart failure) or short-circuiting the electrical system that co-ordinates the heart's pumping mechanism (arrhythmias). In addition, fragments of the fatty deposits in the walls of the vessels may break off and fly to the heart (heart attack) or to the brain (stroke). And it can all be laid at the door of that terrible fat. No wonder the awful stuff has such a bad press.

Nevertheless, a number of studies specifically set up to discover whether a high percentage of body fat correlates with the incidence of coronary heart disease have found no evidence for such a relationship. It has been estimated that increased body mass might produce at most a 5 per cent change in the risk for heart disease across populations – minute in terms of individual risk. Taken in terms of individuals it means that, like the sober drivers having accidents, the *majority of those who develop coronary heart disease are not fat and not overweight.*

There is a slightly stronger association between increasing weight, raised blood pressure and *congestive heart failure*. And it appears that losing weight – at least to begin with – may lower blood pressure (see Caroline's story, pp. 34–5). However, Campos, in *The Obesity Myth*, has collected a vast body of evidence against 'yo-yo dieting' – losing weight and then putting it back on again (more of this in the next chapter), and argues that it is this process which is the real health risk. Obese patients put on very low-calorie diets subsequently experience much higher rates of congestive heart failure than equally fat people who have not attempted to diet.

Something similar has been noted in non-experimental settings. During the Second World War the Germans laid siege to the Soviet city of Leningrad (now St Petersburg) for 900 days from September 1941 to January 1944. Food and fuel gradually ran out. In January 1942, in the depths of an unusually cold winter, food rations in the city were only 125 grams (4 ounces) of bread per day. In January and February 1942, 200,000 people died of cold and starvation. When the siege was lifted and people who had been starving began to recover the weight they had lost, admissions to hospital for hypertension (raised blood pressure) soared by 50 per cent.

Among those who have high blood pressure, the death rate is actually two to three times lower among heavy people compared to those who are underweight. And yet overweight hypertensives are routinely advised to lose weight. Glenn Gaesser comments,

> If a hypertensive obese person follows the advice to lose weight in order to lower blood pressure and the remedy doesn't work (as it often doesn't) then what you have is a weight-reduced hypertensive who is now statistically more likely to die from cardiovascular disease than before.

Type 2 diabetes

This condition is much more common among people who are overweight, and especially those with the Ashwell 'apple' shape with excess adipose tissue round the waist. This is the kind of diabetes that usually, but not invariably, occurs later in life and can normally be controlled without daily doses of insulin. In type 1 diabetes, the body's natural defence mechanism – the autoimmune system – destroys the cells in the *pancreas* that produce insulin. In type 2 the pancreas continues to produce insulin but the body becomes resistant to it.

More people are being diagnosed with type 2 diabetes, and being diagnosed earlier. In fact, children are now occasionally diagnosed with it. The multiple health risks associated with it (heart disease and stroke, damage to kidneys, eyes, nerves, feet, skin) are probably the principal reason why obesity has got such a bad press, by association. These make it very expensive to treat, and the younger people are diagnosed, the longer they will need medication and

monitoring. So when the Cassandras bewailing the dread consequences of the 'obesity epidemic' add the financial cost of fat to the
cost in early death and ill health, their calculations are usually based
on the cost of managing diabetes.

The diagnosis of type 2 diabetes and its warning signs have
increased all over the world in recent years. A study published in the
British Journal of General Practice at the end of 2005 which surveyed
data from 38 general practices for the decade between 1991 and
2001 found a 50 per cent increase in the prevalence. ('Prevalence'
applies cumulatively to all cases of a disease; the number of new
cases each year is the 'incidence'.) To be fair, this does not necessarily mean that twice as many people had type 2 diabetes in 2001
than in 1991. It could also mean that many more had it in 1991 but
were not diagnosed – diabetic 'sleepers'. A great deal of medical
concern has been focused on the disease in recent years and many
cases that were missed before have been identified.

In addition, a group of warning signs that pick up those at risk of
developing the condition has been recognized, known as the metabolic syndrome. Diabetes is a disease of the metabolism: that is, of
the way the body breaks down and uses the raw material in food.
The metabolic syndrome consists of:

- obesity, especially round the abdomen;
- insulin resistance or glucose intolerance, meaning the body cannot use insulin to break down the sugars in food or circulating in
  the blood;
- elevated blood pressure;
- raised levels of 'bad', low-density cholesterol in the blood; the
  kind that contributes to the build-up of fatty plaques in blood-
  vessel walls;
- increased levels of substances that encourage blood clots;
- increased levels of a chemical that signals inflammation.

These symptoms increase the risk of heart attack and stroke, even
without full-blown diabetes, and 80 per cent of people with diabetes
are overweight or obese, although this does not prove that the
excess weight is *causing* the diabetes (they could both be the result
of something else, or the metabolic malfunction of diabetes might

be contributing to the increased weight, rather than the other way round).

Nevertheless, the link between this illness and overweight is more robust than with most other conditions blamed on fat. In controlled animal studies, 50 per cent of monkeys allowed to put on weight developed diabetes. None did so in the group fed a calorie-controlled diet to prevent them putting on weight. A number of long-term studies are under way to see if keeping down the weight of people at risk of type 2 diabetes (those with metabolic syndrome) will prevent them developing the disease, and an initial report suggests that if this can be achieved – and it's a big 'if' – reducing weight can be protective.

So, weighing up the evidence, it appears that much of the hype surrounding overweight and ill health may not be justified. There may be risks with excess fat in particular locations – round the neck or round the tummy – but, to misquote Mark Twain, 'Reports of death from obesity have been greatly exaggerated.' Meanwhile, you might marginally reduce your risk profile by maintaining a stable weight in the mid-range of the BMI, but this is not something everyone can achieve, which leads us to the next chapter.

4

Dieting to lose weight: the good, the bad and the ugly

Let me start by making a distinction: your diet – what you eat – is unquestionably an important factor in being healthy. Diet*ing,* or slimming – eating less, usually with the goal of weighing less – is quite another kettle of fish (or whole grains, fruit and veg or what you fancy). In this chapter, let's look at the evidence for dieting to lose weight being good, bad or extremely bad for your health.

The idea that 'you are what you eat' is as old as the hills and based on some fact, although what people think they can absorb via food is not always well founded. In biblical times, there was a superstitious belief that you could acquire the desirable qualities of an animal – the courage of the lion, the swiftness of the deer – by eating some part of it. These days it's more likely to be some elusive ideal of enhanced health and vitality. However, the idea that you might control your body shape and weight by modifying your diet is relatively recent.

Slimming diets from 1066 and all that

1087   The first person recorded as going on a diet in order to lose weight was William the Conqueror, who grew so fat that he could no longer get up on a horse. Legend has it that he took to his bed and consumed nothing but alcohol. There is no record of how much weight he lost, though it must have had some effect because later in the same year he died as a consequence of falling from his horse. But when they came to bury him he was still so fat they found it virtually impossible to cram him into his coffin.

1733   George Cheyne (see Chapter 1) devises a very modern regime based on exercise, fresh air and a frugal diet, gallons of mineral water, limited alcohol and lots of vegetables which he claims make the body melt away 'like a snowball in summer'. It's worth noting that, in common with dieters the world over, Cheyne's 'snowball' figure returned pretty quickly once the diet was relaxed.

1863 The first slimming publication appears – a short pamphlet called 'Letter on Corpulence Addressed to the Public', a personal case history by a corpulent English undertaker called William Banting. Banting was only 5 feet 7 inches tall, and had weighed 202 pounds for 20 years until a surgeon, whom he consulted about deafness, prescribed a diet which cut out almost all sugar and starch. Banting ate four reasonable meals a day (*'quality* in food is the chief desideratum . . . *quantity* is mere moonshine,' he emphasized) chosen from protein (meat, poultry or fish), green vegetables, unsweetened fruit, several glasses of claret, brandy, gin or whisky, with water and a little dry toast. He ate no root vegetables, potatoes, bread, sugar, sweetened drinks, pastries or desserts. As a result of this precursor of the modern Atkins diet he lost 50 pounds (22.7 kilos) at the rate of about one pound per week – and what's more he stayed at or around his new weight, 11 stone (70 kilos) – for the rest of his days.

1879 The artificial sweetener Saccharin is invented and becomes the basis of chemical giant Monsanto's fortune.

1890s An American doctor called Helen Densmore recommends a diet modelled on Banting from which bread, cereals and starchy foods are excluded: 'One pound of beef or mutton or fish per day with a moderate amount of the non-starchy vegetables will be found ample for any obese person of sedentary habits.' Her patients lost an average of 10 to 15 pounds (4.5 to 6.8 kilos) in the first month and 6 to 8 pounds in each subsequent month. We are not told whether they kept the pounds off.

1896 Commercial weight-loss products start to be advertised. Common ingredients are laxatives, purgatives, arsenic, strychnine, washing soda and Epsom salts!

1918 A new vogue for slimness takes hold and calorie counting is advocated to achieve it. Dr Lulu Hunt Peters publishes a book called *Diet and Health with a Key to the Calories.*

1920s Bathroom scales become a popular phenomenon for monitoring weight. The stars of the new moving pictures carry calorie

reduction to extreme lengths: the Hollywood 18-day diet keeps
people on fewer than 600 calories a day by sticking to citrus fruit,
eggs and Melba toast.

1928   The first clinical dietary trial is set up to test the effects of an
all-protein (meat), no-carbohydrate diet, prompted by the experience
of two arctic explorers, Stefansson and Anderson, who survived on
the Eskimo diet composed exclusively of meat and fish for a number
of years with no apparent ill effects. The experiment lasted a year, and
an eminent medical committee was set up to monitor it and assess its
effect on the volunteers. The results, published in 1930 in the *Journal
of Biological Chemistry*, found that the two men had remained
perfectly healthy.

1932   The first meal substitute, a slimming powder called Dr Stoll's
Diet Aid, is sold through beauty parlours. It contained milk chocolate,
starch, whole-wheat and bran and 22 calories a portion.

1938   The first national slimming organization is established: TOPS
(Take Off Pounds Sensibly). Esther Manz of Milwaukee, USA,
prescribes low calories, scales, food diaries and mutual support for her
members.

1950   The first dieter's cookbook appears: *The Reducer's Cookbook*.
(Copies are still available from second-hand book specialists.)

1963   Weight Watchers founded.

1970s   Dietary concern focuses on reducing the risk of heart disease
and stroke. The Seven Countries Study reveals the effect of variations
in national diet upon the incidence of these diseases. Refined
carbohydrates – sugar and white flour – are identified as the bogey
and dietary fibre is promoted as the good. Government reports link
diet with the incidence of cardiovascular disease (affecting the heart
and circulation) and lay down targets for a reduction in the amount
of *saturated fats*, sugar and salt to be consumed, with an increase in
the amount of fibre.

1982   Audrey Eyton's 'F-Plan' adapts the high-fibre, low-fat diet,
advocated by the medical fraternity for reducing the risk of heart

disease, for slimmers. The book rapidly outsells Penguin Books' previous record-holder, *Lady Chatterley's Lover*. The F-Plan prescribes foods regarded as 'fattening' by low-carb fanatics: wholemeal bread, root vegetables, beans and bran cereals. From now on, new slimming cookbooks and diets hit the headlines with the frequency of new pop-groups. There are diets based on cabbage soup, grapefruit, pickles and apple-vinegar – an aid said to date from Lord Byron's battle with his bulge – all essentially boredom diets that take the fun out of eating.

1992   Banting's low-carb diet (less the alcohol) makes a comeback as Dr Atkins' 'New Diet Revolution', partly due to some very high-profile celebrity slimmers. Between them, his two books sell a total of 16 million copies worldwide. They are joined by Barry Sears' 'The Zone' and the Beverley Hills diet, which last actually allows champagne but not much else. The down-side of pumping the protein and cutting out the carbs begins to emerge. 'It's bad for the kidneys,' say doctors. 'It makes your breath smell,' report the punters.

2000s   Atkins is toppled from its temporary perch by diets based on the *glycaemic index* (GI). This is a way of classifying foods according to how quickly the body breaks them down and converts them into blood sugar, stimulating increased production of insulin. It was first recommended in the 1980s as a way for diabetics to control their insulin levels, and had been popular in Australia for a decade. Doctors support GI diets because at least they include 'complex' carbohydrates like whole grains and high-fibre vegetables, though chocolate and salted peanuts also have a low (good) GI.

Dieting: the good news

Historically, doctors have recommended that patients lose weight for a truly remarkable range of ills and, modern medical experts now agree, not always soundly. These days, dieting is recommended for all the conditions we looked at in the previous chapter and particularly to reduce the risk of cardiovascular disease and type 2 diabetes. If you want a long, vigorous life, it clearly makes sense to adopt behaviour that promotes health and discourages disease. If, as we are given to believe, weight and health are partly inherited and partly the result of environmental triggers and how we cope with them, it seems sensible to modify the second part because it's the only bit over which we have any control.

We live in an age where we are encouraged to take charge of our own lives. We're not always successful, but it's a goal we all pay lip service to, and in developed countries like the UK where society nurtures us from the cradle to the grave we certainly have a lot more autonomy than a peasant in the Middle Ages or an African subsistence farmer.

In fact, losing weight is basically quite easy. You eat less – quite how much less and how long for varies – and ultimately you weigh less. And most people agree: you feel good when you lose weight. Your clothes are looser, you're nimbler, your sex drive increases, and people notice your appearance: 'My word, you do look well.' The 44,000 members who attend Weight Watchers every week, plus all the other dieting clubs, surely can't be wrong.

And, since we are talking about health as well as subjective well-being, losing weight may also reduce your blood pressure, relieve the pressure on arthritic joints, improve your digestion, give you more energy, lower your blood cholesterol, make you sleep better, and improve the way your body responds to insulin if you suffer from the metabolic syndrome. Testimonials from satisfied dieters abound, and our medical advisers urge us on.

So what's the snag? You already know. If the lost weight stayed off, no one would make any money out of it, nor out of diet books or diet aids. Taking off the pounds is not the problem. It's keeping them off. The reason dieting is always on the agenda is that 80 per cent of those who diet put back the weight they have lost, and often put on even more.

(I am unable to verify whether the 80 per cent whose dieting is a failure appear more than once in the statistics – like those much-married people who increase the divorce rate. Is it in fact a slightly smaller percentage of dieters failing again, again and again?)

Dieting that is hazardous to health

Not everyone who tries to lose weight reports a good experience. Many suffer not only hunger pangs – to be expected in the initial stages – but irritability, depression, lethargy and insomnia. They often start to obsess about food, a factor that may lead them to overeat once released from the constraints of dieting. Janet Polivy, a psychologist at the University of Toronto and a specialist in compulsive eating (see her book *Breaking the Diet Habit*) says,

> Dieters are like tightly wound springs – the more restrained their eating, the tighter the spring. Once a dieter goes off his or her diet, the spring releases. The tighter that spring has been wound, the more forceful is its release. The more restrictive the diet, the bigger the binge.

Add together the fact that something like three-quarters of people in the UK or the USA may be dieting at any one time, and the fact that it is spectacularly unsuccessful, and you realize that among the overweight and obese whose health causes the medical establishment such concern there must be numbers of failed or yo-yo dieters. How much does this particular and widespread behaviour contribute to ill health?

A great deal, according to experts like Glen Gaesser, who challenge what they call the 'Diet Mafia' on several fronts. Paul Campos points out that even if a fat person succeeds in losing weight and stays there, it doesn't give him or her the physical characteristics or health profile of someone who is slim naturally. Inside the slim dieter is a fat person trying to get out. Where the yo-yo dieter has been studied independently of those who are stable at above ideal weight, all the indicators are that weight loss is damaging to health.

This is particularly true for the elderly. One study of men and women over 71 found an increased risk of death with a loss as small as 10 pounds (4.5 kilos), even among diabetics, and a 2002 review of 31 trials showed conclusively that weight *gain* in *under*weight old people reduced mortality by about a third. Leading obesity researcher Paul Ernsberger says that no controlled clinical trial (as opposed to an epidemiological one) has demonstrated improved longevity after weight loss, although several have shown it to be correlated with weight gain. Gaesser quotes more than 24 studies over 20 years that demonstrate that weight loss can increase the risk of premature death by a factor of several hundred per cent, primarily from heart disease. (He found four studies that suggested weight loss led to lower mortality, though not by much. Such is the nature of scientific research.) Among the elderly it presents a paradox, as he says, because weight loss is generally thought to improve the risk factors for cardiovascular disease. Gaesser blames the popularity of the low-carbohydrate (Atkins) diet.

Atkins in the frame

Gaesser is not the only expert to deplore the high-protein, low-carb diet for causing a whole range of health problems. The irony is that if weight loss were the only goal there would be no complaint – it demonstrably cuts off the pounds faster than other diets. But this comes at a cost on several fronts. It actually raises the levels of 'bad' (low-density fats) and reduces the 'good' (high-density fats) in the bloodstream. And this, much more than fat on the body, increases the risk of fatty plaques developing in the blood-vessel walls (atheroma) and a general hardening (*atherosclerosis*) which increases the risk of heart attack, stroke and the blocking of the coronary arteries.

Gaesser suggests another reason why weight loss may increase the risk of dying from heart disease. Dieting reduces the body's reserves of healthy *omega-3 fatty acids* which could also make the dieter more vulnerable to atherosclerosis (see Chapter 7).

The Atkins-type diet can also potentially damage the kidneys, the liver and bone formation. To trace the connection, it's necessary to look briefly at the role of carbohydrates and sugars in the diet. You probably already know that carbohydrates, which include sugars, provide energy because they are rapidly absorbed into the bloodstream in the form of blood-sugar, or glucose. Glucose is stored in muscles and in the liver and in the brain as *glycogen*, supplied by carbohydrates in the diet. If you reduce them or remove them from your diet, the body draws upon the stored glycogen. This is what Atkins calls 'fat-burning', or *ketosis*. Glycogen consists of a large number of water molecules, so when it is converted into glucose the body becomes dehydrated. This explains much of the initial weight loss on the Atkins diet, rather than Atkins' claim that the initial weight loss is fat. You can always put back lost fluids (together with lost weight) but the other component of the Atkins diet is lots of protein. Massive amounts of protein, if you are not pregnant, a ballet dancer or a navvy, are not required by the adult body and put extra strain on the kidneys, which in turn leads to a disturbance in the balance of minerals in the body, limiting the kidneys' ability to absorb calcium, which may lead to kidney stones or the early stages of osteoporosis. A study of typical Atkins menus by the University of Kentucky suggested that they might even put the dieter at greater risk of cancer, among other serious risks.

To be fair, it should also be recorded that one study found that a very low-carbohydrate diet was better at improving metabolic syndrome, not surprising when you consider that carbohydrates are the source of glucose in the blood.

But what about the oft quoted improvements in health following weight loss, particularly its effect on raised blood pressure or type 2 diabetes? Ernsberger points out that if people who weigh, say, 300 pounds (136 kilos) were to lose 30 pounds by adopting a diet low on fat and rich in fruit and vegetables, they would still be classified as 'morbidly obese'. So if their blood-sugar, blood pressure and cholesterol all improve, it is clear proof that it is the change of diet that has prompted the change, not their weight. 'Physiologically there is little difference between a 270 pound person maintaining a healthy lifestyle and a 110 pound person . . . Doesn't this prove that it is lifestyle not body fat that is crucial?' he asks. We look at dieting for health rather than weight loss in Chapter 7.

The pharmaceutical dimension

Drugs can make you slim. You only have to look at the emaciated models or pop stars with a cocaine habit. You don't often see a fat alcoholic either. In the past people have swallowed tapeworms or taken insulin when not diabetic as an aid to weight loss. However, no one would claim that this was the route to a healthy weight. But a whole succession of slimming pills have been widely promoted and made fortunes for their manufacturers.

Jerry's story
Jerry had her first baby in the 1960s. A high-powered advertising executive, she had always planned to go back to work after a few months. But she enjoyed breast-feeding and pottering around the flat and playing the housewife, and put on quite a bit of weight in a few months. Then the call came from the agency; they couldn't keep the job open much

longer. Jerry realized that if she was to get into her neat little business suits she would have to slim. The doctor gave Jerry some pills that made her feel energetic and excited and killed her appetite. She rushed round the house like a dervish and the pounds melted like snow in summer. An au pair was engaged and Jerry went back to work. To begin with she kept taking the pills. They gave her such energy. But she began to find it difficult to sleep, had difficulty in concentrating and bashed the car. The doctor found that her blood pressure was going through the roof: she should stop the pills. Jerry felt lethargic and depressed. She was so sleepy that sometimes she put her head on the desk and fell asleep. Jerry had become addicted to amphetamines.

The rise of the diet pill

Folklore apart, the earliest obesity medicine was probably thyroid extract (extracted from sheep's thyroid gland), first tried in the 1880s. It certainly induced weight loss. It put up the rate at which the body produces energy – the metabolic rate. It also put up the blood pressure, gave you diarrhoea and made you feel pretty grotty, but amazingly the treatment, together with the theory 'It's my glands, doctor' became the treatment or explanation for overweight for some 70 years.

Another nasty drug was tried when, in the early 1900s, it was observed that textile workers lost weight after they had inhaled a chemical called dinitrophenol, used to process textiles. The side-effects of this compound were even worse than thyroid extract: it caused cataracts (a thickening of the lens of the eye which clouds vision), nerve damage and even death. It is currently used as a wood preservative and insecticide.

Amphetamines and related drugs were prescribed from the late 1930s. They were issued to pilots and servicemen in the front line during the war to keep them awake, and rumour has it that the US army are still prescribed them in combat zones. This family of drugs is related to cocaine. Its use as a recreational drug has lent it many street names: dexies (short for dextroamphetamine), purple hearts (due to the shape and colour of a popular pill), rainbow pills and speed. It remained a popular drug for weight loss from the 1930s until the 1970s. It is an appetite suppressant, and like most such drugs is potentially addictive, liable to abuse, and certainly not ideal in a population at risk for heart disease. Nevertheless, it continued to be used because it certainly helped people lose weight and, like its bad uncle, cocaine, made users feel gee-ed up and positive – though it also blunted discrimination which made it potentially dangerous for anyone in charge of machinery. Abuse or involuntary addiction became quite a problem and gave obesity medication a bad press from which it has never recovered.

The history of diet pills is riddled with mad enthusiasm followed by shock-horror when unforeseen side-effects emerge. Most, like amphetamines, suppress appetite by working upon neurotransmitters in the brain. They may additionally increase the metabolic rate, raise body temperature and induce wakefulness. Others block absorption (orlistat), or aim to reduce appetite by making you feel full even when you haven't eaten much. Ephedrine, a decongestant long used to treat asthma and present in a number of Chinese herbal treatments, acts on the brain in a way similar to amphetamines. In the 1970s a Danish physician from Elsinore called Eriksen observed that asthmatics on a drug containing ephedrine, caffeine and a barbiturate (an early sedative or sleeping pill) lost weight. Rumour spread about the drug's effect, and when sales reached a peak in 1977, more than 70,000 Danes were said to be taking what became known as the 'Elsinore pill'. A similar combination drug containing ephedrine, known as the Do-Do pill, was available over the counter in England, and it was discovered that the caffeine heightened the heat-producing effect of ephedrine, speeding up the metabolism and thus burning up food faster. A slight variation combining ephedrine and caffeine with aspirin is in the so-called 'ECA stack', a supplement popular with body-builders because it increases energy and alertness.

Fenfluramine and dexfenfluramine were (they have now been withdrawn) two of a group of appetite suppressants that work on the neurotransmitter *serotonin*, like the anti-depressant Prozac. They were used in a range of proprietary drugs. Fenfluramine, combined with a *vasoconstrictor/bronchodilator* (phentermine) also used to treat asthma, became known as Fen-phen and was used for some years in Europe and hailed as a miracle cure for obesity when launched in the United States in 1996. But 18 months later the drug was withdrawn because it was found to cause heart valve problems. Eight diet drugs containing fenfluramine were banned in China following a number of deaths in Asia, and the Open golf champion John Daly attributed a 'mini-stroke' that nearly killed him to diet pills which he had been taking for some time, helping him to lose over two stone. His doctor told Daly, 'You were walking straight into a stroke if you kept taking those pills.'

The last word on diet pills

Paul Campos, in his book *The Obesity Myth*, says of the licensing of fenfluramine by the US Food and Drugs Administration (FDA),

> Rarely, if ever, had a drug with such a long history of dangerous side effects been up for government approval. And for what benefit? The clinical data indicated that dieters taking fenfluramine lost only seven pounds more than dieters taking a placebo . . . It was not a favorable ratio of risk to benefit.

Campos hits the nail squarely on the head by going on to point out that this drug, as well as producing only a tiny weight loss, had not been shown to improve major risk factors associated with high weight, such as high blood pressure and cholesterol. If weight loss, whether by taking pills or even dieting, doesn't improve the health of people who are 'overweight', what's the point of it? The fact is that studies evaluating the effect of diet pills invariably use weight loss as the chief endpoint. They do not include their effect on any of the important health factors mentioned by Campos. Without such information a risk–benefit ratio cannot be established.

Extreme measures

There is one more dramatic way of reducing weight: surgery. Stomach stapling, banding, by-pass or even partial removal is practised in the United Kingdom (where restrictions have recently been placed on its availability on the National Health Service) and the USA as an ultimate solution to extreme and intractable obesity. It is expensive, but makes weight loss pretty inevitable. The rationale behind such extreme and risky procedures is that when a person becomes morbidly obese the health risks pile up and the solutions – especially those involving exercise – become more difficult. (See the box on p. 51, 'Gym bans 21-stone man'.) However, any major open surgical procedure carries risk. In fact, it is often the imminent need for surgery for conditions even more threatening than obesity, like cancer or coronary artery disease, that is the cue for doctors urging the overweight to lose some pounds before they face the knife. To the standard risk of having a general anaesthetic, candidates for weight-loss surgery (known as *gastric banding* or *by-pass)* encounter the additional risk of complications such as wound infection, hernia, dehydration and malnutrition or, more serious but less common, leaks, bleeding and pulmonary embolism. There is a long list of long-term complications. Gastric by-pass carries a 1 in 200 (0.5 per cent) chance of death. Gastric banding, which involves a sleeve or band being slipped round the stomach to narrow it and reduce its capacity, can be carried out with key-hole surgery but still carries a death risk of 1 in 10,000. However, this operation does not notch up such a record of successful weight reduction.

Gym bans 21-stone man

Hospital worker Andy Dowland of Yeovil in south Somerset weighed 21 stone (133 kilos) and was put on a weight-loss programme by his doctor. But when he tried to join his local council-run gym he was turned down as being too 'unfit'. Defending the decision, a council spokesman said that Mr Dowland's blood pressure was dangerously high and that there was a risk that he could suffer a heart attack while using their equipment. Fortunately Mr Dowland managed to find a private gym with a more positive attitude.

Surgical successes

The BBC programme *Inside Out* carried the story of a hugely obese pop singer called Buster Bloodvessel, of the 1980s group Bad Manners. At his heaviest Buster weighed 31 stone (197 kilos), and lost 18 stone (114 kilos) after a novel form of gastric by-pass developed by Professor Michael McMahon at the Leeds Nuffield Hospital. (Several surgeons across the country had refused to operate on Buster for fear he would not survive.) This operation was carried out under the NHS and viewers of *Inside Out* rushed to endorse it (see <http://www.bbc.co.uk/insideout/yorkslincs/series7/buster_bloodvessel.shtml>).

Weight-loss surgery can claim to be an effective means for morbidly obese individuals to lose large amounts of weight and then keep it off, according to a study published in the *Annals of Internal Medicine*, April 2005. Whether they are healthier or just unhealthy in a different way after such an operation is difficult to judge. Gastric by-pass surgery typically results in the loss of 75 per cent of excess weight, and patients only put back on an average of 10 per cent. The loss had been maintained for ten years or longer, so clearly there is a comfortable survival rate. This study also mentions health outcomes: conditions such as sleep apnoea, high blood pressure and type 2 diabetes improved and were frequently eliminated.

With this chapter we come to the end of the examination of the science underpinning health and weight. I am sorry if it has turned out to be rather negative. The price of reassuring those of you who might have felt threatened by talk of obesity epidemics, '300,000 premature deaths' or the urgent necessity of acquiring a BMI of 25 or less, has been that we have claimed that the dangers of being moderately or even severely overweight may have been exaggerated. But I seem to have suggested that there is nothing you can do to improve matters. This is not the case. Unless you are already fantastically healthy and a weight you are happy with – and few are – there are almost certainly things you can do about improving your health and weight. These we will explore in the second part of the book.

Part 2

ACTION

5

Start as you mean to go on

Part 1 of this book was about weighing up the evidence for a connection between weight or fat and health. It was an attempt to sort out hype from sound science, and not an easy task, given that experts do not agree.

The second half of this book concentrates on what you can do to be a healthy weight. Medicine is on notoriously shaky ground when it attempts to give advice on positive health measures. It's much easier to tell people what they shouldn't do! However, having attempted to sort out the prophets of doom ('300,000 extra premature deaths') from the more cautious view ('a healthy weight is the weight someone is when they are healthy') let's go on, undeterred, to assemble advice about how to be, stay or become a healthy weight.

The weight of our children

The key behaviours that shape our lives are learned in childhood: eating behaviour, the foods we like, the activities we enjoy, and patterns of meals and sociable eating, not to mention our acceptance of our own bodies and confidence in our ability to control our lives.

But if your childhood experience in these matters was unfavourable, all is not lost. With confidence and determination, it is possible to teach yourself healthy behaviour and attitudes as an adult. And, on the assumption that many of us are parents, I would like to start with how to give children the best start, because the medical angst about obesity in adults is nothing to the chorus of disapproval raised about the phenomenon of obesity in children.

Overweight children were once considered unusual and abnormal, but in countries all over the world they are becoming increasingly common. It's happening not just in the developed world – including the USA, the UK and Australia – but also in developing countries:

Brazil, Chile, Haiti, Ghana, Morocco, Egypt and even China and Japan, where for generations the people were naturally and effortlessly slim. Population studies do not, as we have remarked already, all use the same yardstick of overweight (the standard BMI is not suitable for assessing children); nevertheless, several have examined prevalence over an interval of time and their results are 'astounding', to quote the medical journal *The Lancet* in a 2002 seminar on the issue of childhood obesity. In England, rates have more than doubled over ten years. In the USA they have increased more than threefold in about 25 years, and in Egypt nearly fourfold over 18 years. The heaviest children – those at risk of complications – have become even heavier, and the phenomenon affects children of all ages and ethnic and socioeconomic groups, although in America prevalence rose twice as fast in minority groups compared with whites, exacerbating pre-existing racial-ethnic disparities in health. *The Lancet* questions whether the poor in developed countries (the UK and the USA) may not be particularly at risk because of poor diet and a sedentary lifestyle, although the report notes that in the developing nations it is more common among the rich, where over-nutrition and under-nutrition coexist, possibly due to the tendency to adopt a Western lifestyle and diet.

Before birth

Genetic factors apart, the environmental factors that affect health and weight start in the womb. In 1989 a British doctor called David Barker noticed a relationship between an elevated death rate among newborn babies in one impoverished region of the UK in the 1900s and a high incidence of heart disease in the same area decades later. This presented a paradox, because at this time heart disease was considered to be a disease of affluent people leading inactive, stress-ridden lives on a high-fat diet, whereas high neonatal mortality was recognized as a sign of poverty. Perhaps, he thought, a predisposition to heart disease might be caused *not* by a combination of genes and adult behaviour alone, but also by the foetal experience in the mother's womb. He found support for this hypothesis in other historical records. Mothers who had conceived in occupied Europe during the Second World War while existing on starvation rations had had babies who had been small at birth, become fat during childhood and developed heart disease or type 2 diabetes (closely associated with obesity) as adults.

David Barker's research is described in Chapter 2, and also in his book *Mothers, Babies and Health in Later Life*. The pattern he observed was one of poor nutrition in the womb, leading to low birth weight followed by exceptional, and atypical for normal development, weight gain between the ages of 2 and 11, and coronary heart disease and type 2 diabetes in adulthood. He postulated a 'thrifty metabolism' that had developed in response to undernourishment in the womb but which was inappropriate in the face of adequate or abundant nutrition in childhood.

Several studies have supported Barker's hypothesis and attempted to explain it. Recently Japanese researchers, working with mice, reported in the journal *Cell Metabolism* that a premature surge of the hormone leptin (looked at in Chapter 2) led to a reprogramming of key brain circuits that control appetite and metabolism, and contributed to obesity in the animals later in life.

Other researchers have advanced the idea that obesity might also be caused by *over*-nutrition in the womb and have pointed to a direct relationship between obese mothers, high birth weight and obesity in the offspring later in life. It certainly happens with rats and the phenomenon can be observed in humans. But the impossibility of unravelling the contribution made by inherited genes and family behaviour makes the influence of nutrition in the womb difficult to quantify. Obesity is also more common among children who were bottle-fed rather than breast-fed.

Health complications of childhood obesity

Does it matter if more children are fat? Does it mean that they are also unhealthy? Evidence is emerging that some of the symptoms that pave the way to illness in later life are occurring earlier and earlier, especially in obese children. The potential complications of obesity in childhood are listed in *The Lancet* seminar. They are depressingly familiar. The usual cluster of factors associated with cardiovascular disease – elevated blood fats, raised blood pressure, increased tendency to produce blood clots, and insulin resistance, the so-called metabolic syndrome – has been identified in children as young as five years old. The blood vessels of adolescents who have died of other causes have shown all the symptoms of serious cardio-vascular disease, with fatty plaques in blood-vessel walls (atheroma) particularly pronounced in those who were obese. In one group of British children, being overweight in childhood doubled the risk of dying of heart disease as an adult up to the age of 57 years. Breathing difficulties, asthma and resistance to doing exercise are other frequent complications which, as with adults, make things worse by restricting healthy activity. Type 2 diabetes, which used to be unknown in children and teenagers, now accounts for as many as half of all new diagnoses of diabetes in some populations.

The report says the increase is 'almost entirely attributable' to the increase in childhood obesity, though it acknowledges the role played by inherited or lifestyle (poor diet and lack of physical activity) factors. And in addition to all these health risks, overweight children also have a tough time at school and often get bullied or teased, leading to poor self-esteem and depression.

All the usual suspects

You can imagine what most experts, including *The Lancet*, blame for this sorry state of affairs: junk food, too little time spent on the playing fields and too much in front of the telly munching fatty snacks and guzzling fizzy drinks. And there are persuasive studies that support this 'ain't it awful' view of modern life. In one, published in the *Journal of the American Medical Association* in 1999, Thomas Robinson compared a group of children who cut back their television viewing by 40 per cent with a control group who continued to view as much as they liked. In the control group, BMI, skinfold thickness on the arm, and waist and hip circumferences all increased significantly, and cardio-respiratory fitness went down, but the group with the reduced viewing lost weight and showed comparable improvements in other health measures. The study was part of an ongoing research programme at Stanford University, California, examining the negative effects of television viewing on children's health and behaviour.

The link between the increased consumption of unhealthy snack foods and television viewing, and between childhood obesity and television viewing at mealtimes, is also supported by research. Comparable studies have looked at the impact of fewer hours' physical education in schools, the selling off of school playing fields, the loss of public parks and streets suitable for playing in and, of course, the rise and rise of the motor car as the preferred mode of transport, especially to and from school. Beneath this anxiety-promoting research, and more particularly the media reporting of such studies, is an underlying fear of change and modernity. Did medieval parents bemoan the tendency for children who should be out hewing wood or drawing water to bury their heads in these new-fangled books? Certainly the advent of mass-circulation newspapers, moving pictures, even the humble bicycle – each, in its turn, has been heralded as the end of civilization as we know it and the downfall of our children. Heed a word of warning from sceptics Michael Gard and Jan Wright in *The Obesity Epidemic*: 'It is a truism that there is a human tendency for each generation to despair about the generation that follows it.'

A similar tendency to see the harmful present in relation to a notional golden age informs much of the reporting on the limitations of present-day children's diet. Here sound evidence exists, but it is important to sift out the genuinely harmful from the merely faddy. There is evidence, for example, that we are consuming more so-called snack or junk food, both at home, in take-away foods and in restaurant meals, and in Chapter 7 we will look at what it is about such foods that makes them not conducive to 'healthy weight'. The indictment is particularly strong against sugary soft drinks. A study of a group of American schoolchildren, also reported in *The Lancet*, observed a 60 per cent increased risk of becoming obese for every additional daily serving consumed. A controlled study with English primary school children, reported in the *British Medical Journal*, was carried out to see if reducing the consumption of these drinks would lead to a reduction in obesity. After a year, the number of obese children in the intervention group had gone down by only a 'modest' 0.2 per cent. However, in the control group of unfettered pop-guzzlers the percentage that was obese had actually increased by 7.5.

The Lancet 2002 seminar reviews a number of US interventional school programmes, only one of which, 'Planet Health', run by Harvard Prevention Research, had had much success, and then only with girls. The programme aimed at improving the diet, increasing physical activity, limiting television viewing and reducing the incidence of obesity, and its success with the girls was attributed to a reduction in their television viewing.

The Lancet authors conclude that most interventional approaches have been 'disappointing', although a few family-based programmes had had some success in producing long-term weight loss in people who were truly motivated. Let us now progress to suggesting some of the things that may achieve this desirable state of affairs.

Prevention is better than cure, example better than instruction

Children, unlike adults, spend many years of their lives as guests at others' tables. They eat meals provided by parents, schools and friends, and maybe by the local take-away or McDonald's. This puts the food-providers in a position of considerable influence. They should use it responsibly to educate children in making intelligent, discriminating choices about food that will equip them to deal sensibly with the seductions that assail them all around, and above all to avoid food as comfort. Food can be many things apart from nourishment. It can be sociability, aesthetic pleasure, achievement – when you produce or cook it yourself – but once it becomes comfort it risks being used inappropriately, excessively or even harmfully.

Where food choice is concerned, the best option is for parents to propose and children to dispose; in other words, offer them interesting, nourishing and varied food but for heaven's sake let them choose from these. Never either compel or (totally) deny. One other general principle: you must lead by example. It is hopeless to suggest children avoid nibbling between meals if you are always resorting to the biscuit barrel; or that they take strenuous exercise unless you go with them on a brisk hike or bike ride. Fortunately children occasionally amaze you by failing to imitate your bad behaviour. (One of the things that made me a life-long, committed non-smoker was all the horrid little containers of ash my mother used to litter the house with.)

If you can follow these guidelines you may prevent your children ever putting on too much weight in the first place, and it's so much easier to avoid extra weight than to take it off later. You won't prevent your teenage daughter developing rather heavy thighs if it runs in the family, nor can you prevent your adolescent son being skinny, gangly and quite incapable of controlling his limbs when he hits the growth spurt, if that build is also in his genes. You are not bringing up children to be catwalk models: you are trying to help them achieve and maintain the weight and shape that is natural and comfortable for them.

Babies

Given that during pregnancy you keep a careful eye on your diet and your weight, you will ensure you have your folic-acid supplement, abjure the booze, and eat a balanced diet in slightly greater quantities than before becoming pregnant.

In an ideal world, once the baby arrives, you will breast-feed. I know: some women say they 'can't get started'; others say it hurts, or worry that their baby is not getting enough nourishment, but in the days before Monsieur Nestlé and Mr Cow and Gate made themselves a fortune, all babies were breast-fed, albeit not always by their mothers. Babies can, of course, become happy and healthy even if not breast-fed. But breast-feeding is such a wonderful start for mother and baby. It cements the bond. It's hygienic; it's formulated to suit the baby's underdeveloped digestive system; and when you come to evaluate the health outcomes, breast is indisputably best. The health risks to the bottle-fed baby include not only a greater chance of developing obesity in childhood, but an increased risk of insulin-dependent diabetes (type 1), asthma and eczema, and significantly more middle-ear infections, respiratory, intestinal and other bacterial infections. Some studies even suggest that they turn out to be less bright than their breast-fed siblings. Quite apart from the perfect formulation of breast milk, the bond that feeding sets up between mother and child, and the ease of doing it when you are half asleep at three in the morning, the act of sucking on a nipple as opposed to a synthetic teat is beneficial to the development of the roof of the baby's mouth and makes it less likely to swallow air, or to gulp down too much milk. But if you can't breast-feed, it's not the end of the world. You can still establish good eating habits when a toddler is weaned on to the beginning of an adult diet.

Toddlers

If there are two inborn attributes that cement the bond between parent and child more than any other, they are a good digestion and an inclination to sleep through the night. Some fussy babies become picky toddlers, and this can make for anxious mealtimes while the infant's weight is being monitored regularly for developmental progress. Books are available that deal with this problem in detail. Here I will say only that at this formative age it is really important not to let feed-times develop into a battleground. It is unlikely a normal, healthy baby will fade away through undernourishment, and one thing is certain: babies will certainly not eat too much. Keep mealtimes enjoyable at all costs. If they leave one thing, try them with another – healthy option, of course. Beware of using the sweet snack as a reward for finishing the mashed carrot. It helps to establish the sociable nature of mealtimes if you bring the high-chair to the table and talk to the baby, as you do to each other.

Three to six

In early childhood a child's body mass normally decreases until about five to six years, then increases through to adolescence. At this age, children can be trusted to pace their own food consumption to match their energy needs. The parent's goal is to establish good eating habits and healthy attitudes to food. Here are a few guidelines.

- Give children some choice, but not too much.
- Allow children to say how much they want but never force them to finish food. Many overweight adults and also anorexics blame their problem on being forced to eat as children.
- Provide variety but don't worry if they develop preferences.
- Discuss food and their preferences with them, though not obsessively. Encourage them to savour food and express appreciation

when they like it. Discrimination requires cultivation, and good cooking flourishes with praise.

- Never let children eat alone or in front of the television or carry on with any other activity during meals, except talking to one another. Sit with them and have a drink even if you are not eating with them.
- Spend time preparing meals. In the 1960s it took about two and a half hours to prepare a meal; these days popping a ready-meal into a microwave takes minutes. In France 76 per cent of meals are prepared and eaten at home, and the French have less of a problem with overweight than either the British or the Americans.
- Make meals something of an occasion. Lay the table attractively and get the children to help. Cultivate the art of conversation, and have discussions which the children can join in. It slows down eating and illustrates that meals are more than refuelling.
- Encourage children to cook. It can be fun, even if it leaves the kitchen in a mess.
- Grow something with them, even if it is only cress. Growing and cooking are pleasures quite distinct from eating food.
- If you eat out or buy a take-away, encourage experiment.
- However, if your child chooses to exist on a diet of tuna and sweet-corn for a few months, don't worry. He or she will grow out of it.
- Discourage eating between meals. If they must, give them fruit, not sweets or biscuits.
- If they crave sweets or chocolate, ration them: only at certain times or only on certain occasions and always in limited quantities. Never give sweets as rewards or to keep them quiet.
- The same goes for McDonald's and the dreaded hamburger. Do not deny them totally, but ration the visits and encourage children to experiment with different, better-balanced restaurant meals.

At this age, one thing you probably don't need to worry about is making sure they get enough exercise. Persuading them to be sedentary occasionally is more of a problem.

Many of these guidelines carry forward to the later years. The difference from the age of five is that school food, the pressure of peers and the temptations relayed via television become factors in their eating.

School days

From the moment a two-year-old first learns to say 'No' a parent has to face up to losing more and more control. You cannot control everything they do, or protect them from all the hazards and temptations that surround them. Your best hope is to teach them how to look after themselves. This becomes particularly true once they go to school. 'Harry's mummy gives him crisps and chocolate. Why do I have to have fruit and a chicken sandwich?' 'It was spaghetti and chips again at lunch today.' If the notorious Turkey Twizzlers feature too frequently on the school menu you can, of course, persuade your children to take a packed lunch, as long as you are sure they will not be eating it in unsociable isolation. If you have established some good habits before they face school lunches, they could even prove a useful exercise in discrimination and send them home ravenous to eat a huge, healthy supper, rather than acquire a life-long penchant for spaghetti and chips. You could also try inviting Harry and other friends home, where you are in charge of the healthy catering, and you might even get Harry interested.

In their book *Help Your Child Get Fit Not Fat*, Jan Hurst and Sue Hubberstey provide a list of useful tips for composing a healthy but appealing lunch-box, but they point out that parents alone cannot improve the nutritional quality of school food. The government must accept some responsibility. (In the light of the mean sum allocated towards school food by some education authorities, revealed during Jamie Oliver's 'School Dinners' campaign, it's not so surprising what gets served up.) Hurst and Hubberstey comment favourably on the introduction of Breakfast Clubs, which has done much to overcome children's resistance to this important start to the day and to encourage the important social nature of meals, and say that the free fruit schemes in nurseries and primary schools are having some effect, although it will be up to parents to sustain the habit when the levels of expenditure currently allocated are withdrawn.

What about exercise at this age? Many children no longer play hopscotch in the street, schools in England have been selling off their playing fields for development with careless abandon, and fewer and fewer children are getting the daily hour of physical exercise recommended by the World Health Organization. The Department of Education's endlessly reformulated 'national curriculum' is so focused upon tests and targets for academic attainment that physical education in schools has slipped way down the agenda. At the moment only two hours a week are recommended, and some schools are not even managing this. Hurst and Hubberstey quote a director of the Children's Play Council who claims that in a single generation the 'home habitat' of a typical eight-year-old – the area in which children are able to travel on their own – has shrunk to one-ninth of its former size.

This is not just down to reduced activity *in* school. Thirty or more years ago it was quite common for children to cycle or walk several miles to school. These days they are more likely to be transported in a fleet of four-by-fours. This change is usually put down to parents' justifiable fear of traffic and less justifiable fear of 'stranger danger'. (The murder rate of children has not risen, and anyway, nearly 90 per cent of child victims *know* their abuser.) On the principle that parents cannot protect their children in all situations but, more wisely, enable their children to protect themselves, it might be better, not to mention healthier, to teach them how to negotiate heavy traffic at an early age, rather than ferrying them everywhere in a car. The highest rate of child traffic accidents occurs in children over 11, the age when they are most likely to start going to school on their own. This mirrors the high accident rate of inexperienced drivers. Lack of practice and training is what makes people vulnerable, at any age.

Well-meaning relatives – grandparents, a former partner or a step-parent – may also make unwelcome inroads on your attempts to encourage healthy eating. Pampering and providing treats is a natural way of cementing relationships that are occasional rather than live-in, and when this takes the form of sweets or other energy-laden goodies that are frowned on at home you run the risk of being seen as a kill-joy if you make attempts to prevent it. In this situation your safest bet may be to ensure that the fond relative (or competitive ex and partner) know what treats and rewards your children crave that are *not* fattening – like going bowling or shopping for books or DVDs – but which are just as good as a demonstration of affection.

Troubled teens

It is probably more difficult to play a positive role in helping your children maintain a healthy weight once they hit their teens than at any time before. Anxiety about their physical appearance peaks in both sexes, but particularly the girls. As their hormone production surges they may get fatter or thinner without any obvious change in their eating habits, or they may justifiably develop a bigger appetite to fuel their physical growth. Attempts to influence them are interpreted as interfering, and there is a strong urge to rebel against parental rules or patterns of behaviour just to demonstrate how independent and grown-up they now are.

Rachel's story

Rachel's parents were Polish Jews who had emigrated to England before the Second World War. Her father worked as a tailor; her mother was a housewife with inordinate pride in her cooking. Rachel became something of a star at school and they were both inordinately proud of her too. 'They couldn't have been more supportive,' said Rachel. 'But I couldn't share my interest in Shakespeare or Keats with them and I think my mother in particular felt devalued as I got more and more involved with school work and my friends. Her way of showing her affection was constantly urging me to eat huge, fatty, meaty meals. They had experienced the Warsaw ghetto, and that's what she believed growing children needed.'

At 13 Rachel began to put on weight and decided to become a vegetarian. Both her parents were quite plump. 'I really did get hung up about cruelty to animals,' she said, 'but I think it was partly a defence against the endless soups and stews.' Mealtimes became a battleground. Rachel's mother couldn't understand anyone not wanting meat. And anyway, she thought a few curves in a woman were very right and proper. Rachel stuck to her guns and gradually her weight came under control. 'But my mother never really forgave me. Now when I go home I am presented with the groaning board laden with rich food. I tell her I'm not hungry, and she feels unloved.'

As the parent of a teenager you have probably got to resign yourself to the fact that your place is in the wrong. Nevertheless, here are a few helpful guidelines that may enable you to escape their scathing scorn or resentment now, and earn you grudging appreciation later in life.

- Never comment critically on their appearance: their figures, their skin or most especially their choice of clothes or hairstyle. They are discovering their adult identity and are allowed to make a few blunders along the way – and anyway, it's rude to make personal remarks.

- Never praise the appearance of their friends, nor especially any celebrity or pop star on television, in front of them. It may be seen as veiled criticism and will also encourage them to emulate the looks of others, especially the exceptionally thin. If you are asked (not unless) point out that people come in all shapes and sizes and that not only the slim and pretty are attractive, and that fashions in body shape are always changing. Marilyn Monroe was a size 16 and drop-dead gorgeous.

- Ban the subject, the very word, 'diet', even if you secretly indulge yourself. Some parents hide the bathroom scales, but this may be a little extreme. Studies done in the USA suggest that dieting in childhood, especially before the age of 14, may permanently upset the body's metabolism and increases the likelihood of being obese as an adult.

- Praise their appearance, but in moderation. Make sure you also praise them for their achievements, originality, humour and kindness. It is vital not to give girls the impression that it is only their looks that get them attention.

- Encourage them to take exercise, but in a low-key way. Many girls take against school sport in their teens, especially if they feel their new breasts bouncing about when they play, but they may enjoy a dance class. Hopefully some boys will continue playing games, but if they don't, try and find them a non-competitive activity like swimming or riding. Ideally establish a family habit of cycling, bowling or long walks which are fun as well as being good for you.

- Be careful how you react to their emergent sexuality. Never make uninvited comments on chin-fuzz or breast buds, but be prepared to talk naturally and frankly to them if they want to discuss anything. Some parents, dads in particular, feel subconsciously threatened by teenage sexuality; they want their babies to stay that way. It is important that teenagers learn to accept the adult changes in their bodies. Anorexia may be spurred by a rejection of the mature body.

I hope this rather cosy scenario doesn't give you the impression that keeping children happy and a healthy weight in their teens is simple. It's not. You are losing control of them, so you may as well get used to the idea. You may do all the sensible things we recommend and still one of them will get chubby and become unhappy about it. Comfort them with the thought that a slim figure is not everything in life, and that if the weight persists despite a healthy lifestyle they were probably designed to be that way. Only if a child gets really seriously obese – say 20 to 25 per cent heavier than most of their age-group – should you think of suggesting he or she talk to your doctor. On no account ever put a child on a reducing diet without professional advice.

6

Avoiding or limiting weight gain

OK, so dieting to lose weight is bad for you and doesn't work anyway. You are not one of those who can eat what they like and stay thin as a rake. You want to be healthy and keep active but not get too fat. What do you do? A common pattern, varied in how it is implemented, goes by the trade name of chronic restrained eating (CRE). It appears to be the hallmark of successful weight control.

Martin's story
Martin is 5 feet 6¾ inches – 'don't forget the three-quarters' – or 1.7 metres. Once he realized that he was not going to get any taller he also determined not to get any broader. His mother is even shorter (and fatter), as was his father, who died of a heart attack in his sixties. Martin plans to live longer. He swims; he rides his bike to and from the uni, where he works, and he only drinks beer at the weekends. He enjoys his food, but when he finds his 'test' trousers getting a bit tight he clears out the fridge of everything except eggs and apples. 'I call it the boredom diet,' he says. Many famous diets mimic the concept. 'It works fine when I am single, but if I am with someone who cooks for me I weaken,' he says.

Andrea's story
Andrea's mum was slim, but smoked like a chimney; Dad was short and sturdy, with a tendency to fat round the tum. Andrea is also muscular and big-boned and was always heavier than her class-mates at school; then, in her teens, she shot up to 11 stone (70 kilos). Andrea wanted to be an actress so she decided she would have to slim. She noted down what she was eating, cut it down, and lost weight. At drama school controlled eating was easy. In a bedsit on a tiny grant she couldn't afford any luxuries and she cycled everywhere. 'Mum gave me fruit and vegetables from the garden when I went home, but apart from that I lived on milk and cereal.' The discipline became second nature and stood her in good stead in later life. 'I wasn't just chronically restrained as an eater. I was a chronically restrained spender too. I budget food just as I do money, or my time. I enjoy seeing how far I can spread

things. I never put on much more than four pounds; when I do, I cut back a little until I'm back to my fighting weight. I like to be in control of things.'

Neil's story
Unlike the other case histories in this book where I have changed names and distinguishing details for confidentiality, I can reveal Neil Grigg's identity because in 2001 he featured in a front-page story in *USA Today*. For 20 years Neil, a 61-year-old professor of civil engineering, 5 feet 11 inches tall (1.8 metres), had maintained a weight of 190 pounds (about 86 kilos) by limiting his daily food intake to 2,100 calories, walking several miles a day and doing weights. He had discovered exactly what it took to achieve this goal in a scientific laboratory, and every day he jots down the calorie content of what he plans to eat. He eats only the best, and if something he is fond of is calorie-rich, like ice-cream, he eats only a small one, and not too often. *USA Today* hailed the professor and those like him beneath a headline: 'There is a way to keep off the weight', and went on to describe CRE which is, said the author, Nanci Hellmich, not a diet but 'a general philosophy about food'.

The depressing stories about dieting speak repeatedly about the 70–80 per cent of weight regained. But what about those who succeed either in not gaining or in losing and keeping it lost? What distinguishes them? Would anyone ever try to control their weight if there were no evidence of rewarding success? When you start to talk to those who have succeeded or – just as important – have accepted what is achievable for them, you discover that there are any number of ways to arrive there. What all CREs have in common with Martin, Andrea and Neil is that they are highly motivated, have confidence in themselves – a confidence that is boosted by their success – and haven't let their weight spiral out of control. People *can* become CREs after massive weight gain, but they are more frequently those for whom a 10 or 15 per cent weight loss is enough to make them feel comfortable with themselves, or they are people who have never allowed their weight to increase more than, say, seven pounds.

Who dares, wins

This is why slimming organizations try to keep a record of their successes – to encourage others. The risk is that such records are self-selective: those who relapse drop off the record, and only those on course stay in touch. In the USA the National Weight Control Registry (NWCR, <http://www.nwcr.ws/>) was set up to identify and investigate the characteristics of people who succeed in long-term weight loss, who have lost at least 30 pounds (13.6 kilos) and kept it off for at least six years. Detailed questionnaires and annual follow-up surveys are used to examine the behavioural and psychological characteristics of these successful weight-losers and weight-maintainers, and the strategies they use to achieve this. The study has been running since 1994 and now has records for more than 5,000 adults. They have a number of stratagems in common.

- They exercise regularly; walk an average of four miles a day or take some other form of physical activity.
- They limit their calories intake to an average of about 1,800 a day.
- They follow a low-fat diet for health and never skip breakfast.
- They weigh themselves regularly: how regularly varies.
- They eat consistently. (Their diet is not binge and fast; it is a maintenance diet.)
- They keep track of what they eat.

The NWCR was founded in 1993 by medical researchers Rena Wing from Brown Medical School and James O. Hill from the University of Colorado. The results of their ongoing studies of those on the Registry have contributed the bullet points above. Other interesting findings include that the longer weight loss was maintained, the easier it became; successful 'slimmers' also used fewer weight maintenance strategies and found that less attention was required to maintain weight. Loss-maintainers also suffered less distress, depression and loss of energy than those who regained weight who also, unsurprisingly, had a stronger urge for the occasional binge.

In one of their most recent studies Wing and her colleagues used what they had learned about successful weight control from the Registry to evaluate the most effective kind of social support. They had already learned that daily weighing, exercise for at least 30 minutes a day and putting on the brakes when about five pounds were regained, were characteristic of successful weight maintenance. So they recruited people who had lost 10 per cent or more of their body weight over two years in a variety of ways, then allocated them to three support groups – via a newsletter, via the Internet or via a face-to-face support group – to see which group would be most successful in implementing the signal behaviours. In the newsletter group 70 per cent exceeded the five-pound regain threshold, as did just over half the Internet group, but only 38 per cent of those in the face-to-face support group. The amount of weight gained was in parallel: ten pounds for the newsletter group, six for the Internet group and two and a half for the face-to-face group. Of those who stuck to daily weighing, more than 60 per cent gained less than five pounds. As expected, the most successful also stuck to the half-hour daily exercise. The researchers concluded that the face-to-face programme was the most successful because those attending got useful tips on how to modify their eating and exercise behaviour in response to small weight gains. (For case histories, see the NWCR website.)

Changing your relationship with food

These days *cognitive behaviour therapy* (CBT) is being recommended for every problem under the sun, so why not weight loss and loss maintenance? LighterLife is one commercial British weight-loss programme that claims greater recorded success than many other face-to-face groups. Founded in 1996, it has presented studies validating the programme at international conferences and in the *Journal of Obesity*. The organization has tracked 135 subjects for three years, during which time no one regained weight in the first year, and at most 10 per cent of weight lost had been regained after three years. LighterLife is a weight-loss programme for those who want to lose at least three stone (19 kilos), although it also offers a weight-maintenance programme. It's basically a 'boredom diet' and no different from Dr Stoll's Diet Aid (see Chapter 4) in that it depends, at least in the weight-loss phase, on nutritionally balanced, calorie-controlled 'foodpacks' – liquid shakes, soups and bars – instead of real food.

Where the programme is distinctive is in allocating each dieter to a counsellor trained in CBT techniques and/or *transactional analysis* (a form of psychotherapy that works via the relationship established between patient and counsellor to change the subject's relationship with others or their environment, in this case food and eating). CBT aims to modify a person's thought patterns and, via these, their behaviour. LighterLife's co-founder Bar Hewlett says,

> We treat obesity as a form of addiction. This means that first you have to learn to do without food completely, and then – because no one can live on foodpacks indefinitely – how to negotiate food in a moderate and controlled way. We aim to change people's relationship with food so that they no longer see it as reward, comfort, or as love. Rewards, and we encourage people to reward themselves when they reach their goals, are non-food treats – a CD, something to wear, a visit to the theatre. Since many people who put on weight also have low self-esteem we also try to increase self-confidence – giving them confidence to take control of eating and taking exercise – and self-acceptance – because losing weight does not mean that you automatically acquire the figure of a pop star or a model. At the last count success is measured not just in how much you lose but in becoming happy with your own body.

The French have a perfect phrase for this: *'Etre bien dans sa peau.'* It means to be happy in your own skin, and we will return to the concept later in the chapter.

Is endless vigilance a reasonable price to pay for controlling your weight?

People who existed on three 500 calorie LighterLife foodpacks a day admit frankly that they were starving, and often nauseous with it at the start. This distress which inevitably accompanies any sudden reduction of food intake attracts the disapproval of obesity researcher Paul Ernsberger, who puts the question slightly differently: 'Is it better to live fat than to die thin and malnourished?' So let's be clear: neither Martin, Andrea, Neil, nor any of the LighterLife success stories is either thin or malnourished. Far from it.

Chapter 4 examined the health risks most frequently attributed to gaining weight and came to the conclusion that they were not as severe as had been claimed. Paul Campos in *The Obesity Myth* is at pains to remind us that the apocalyptic scare stories about a 'fat epidemic' hanging over us like the sword of Damocles for more than 20 or 30 years have 'so far failed to produce any visible effect on overall life expectancy – other than to correlate nicely with its increase'. We are still at risk of osteoarthritis, raised blood pressure and even type 2 diabetes if we keep a steady, healthy weight into middle age, albeit a slightly lower risk. So is CRE worth the effort?

It depends on your viewpoint. Campos clearly thinks not. He calls CRE 'a life-time sentence', and suggests that in adopting it 'you eat less than you want to eat, and little or none of many of the foods you would most like to eat, almost every day for the rest of your life'. He speaks of 'several decades of daily denial', or

> spending hours every day in what CRE enthusiasts describe as a state of 'constant vigilance' planning and calculating the caloric damage of every meal well ahead of time, agonizing about whether today is the day that one can allow a morsel of brownie to pass one's lips or whether one will be able to resist temptation at the salacious wedding buffet.

Campos here reveals something very important about his attitude to weight control. He has dieted all his life, and it hurts. For Campos self-denial is pain. And he's not alone, as Harry's story shows.

Harry's story
Harry is a GP in Wales. To his patients and friends he seems happy, healthy, positive and average-sized, though not thin – a fine figure of a man. But Harry is a secret CRE. Only his wife realizes the discipline that keeps him the way he is, and the price he pays. 'Both of my parents and all my cousins were morbidly obese,' he confides; 'I wake up hungry and am hungry all day until I go to sleep. So I expend a lot of energy keeping to the shape I am.'

He started controlling his weight as a schoolboy – at 12 he was 'podgy'. His teachers encouraged him to take up running, and he has kept it up for 50 years. Without exercise four days a week, he puts on weight. And without CRE he balloons. Once, on his honeymoon, he relaxed: disaster – he gained three stone! Forty years on he is not quite his pre-marriage weight, but he has at least stayed steady and just over 12 stone. But the constant desire to eat more than he needs has never left him.

Fortunately some have a better experience. Listen to Andrea on the same theme, controlled living:

> I get a kick out of being in control. I plan my time in order to cram in as much as I can. I budget on the same principle: planning makes a little money go further – you spend on those things that really matter. You

don't fritter it away on impulse purchases. I apply the same principle to food. I eat those things that I enjoy and that keep me healthy, but I eat them in quantities that leave me in charge of what I weigh. Discipline is not constraint.

In the passage that I quote opposite from *The Obesity Myth*, Campos' cool determination to excise the hype from the claims of obesity researchers appears to desert him. He makes statements unsubstantiated by research or even anecdote. He is clearly moved by deep feeling. Of course, some people do suffer from not being able to buy on impulse as much as not being able to eat on impulse. Such people may never be able to separate themselves from craving more. 'I have no satiety mechanisms,' my father used to say as he helped himself to another piece of cake, ' – though sometimes I decide to stop.' But who is the more obsessed? The person who plans what they eat or the person who sees saying 'No' to food occasionally as 'decades of daily denial'?

CRE doesn't have to require endless calorie counting. All the practitioners I spoke to said that after time the pattern become instinctive, just what is reported by those on the National Weight Loss Registry, but something Campos believes Americans to be incapable of. Martin's 'test' trousers, Andrea's bathroom scales ('I don't do it daily; because weight goes up and down all the time by a pound or so, but weekly') are like an alarm clock: an occasional reminder to alert them to action; to their modified personal eating plan until they have returned to what they regard as their healthy weight.

Body image and self-confidence are the key

Perhaps my own bias also shows in this chapter. I own up to being a CRE, though I didn't know what it was called until I started researching the book. There is so much failure and gloom in the statistics concerning weight control that it was gratifying to discover that someone had identified a distinct, if small, group of people able to control their weight and that the characteristics that distinguished them had been noted and studied. At Stanford University of Medicine in California, researchers studied a small (177) group of men and women, mildly or moderately overweight, assigned to one of two alternative weight-loss programmes with the goal of picking out any physiological, behavioural, psychosocial or demographic variables that might distinguish the successful from the unsuccessful. They discovered, not surprisingly, that although those on the diet-plus-exercise programme tended to lose slightly more weight than those on the diet-only programme – and they didn't set the bar very high: two units of body mass over a year – the real distinction was in their attitudes and previous experience. Those who started the experiment more satisfied with their bodies and who, in addition, had no history of repeated weight loss and regain – the dreaded yo-yo dieting – were most likely to succeed (63 per cent in the diet-plus-exercise programme). Those who were dissatisfied with their bodies and/or had a history of yo-yo dieting had a greater risk of failure whichever programme, diet-plus-exercise or diet-only, they followed; only 36 and 25 per cent succeeded.

The importance of a history of yo-yo dieting is familiar. It probably reduces the metabolic rate and it certainly teaches sufferers to anticipate failure, never a good starting point. But the psychological factors identified are particularly significant. Several other studies support the finding that a positive body image is a good predictor of dieting success, and that dieters' perception of success – in other words, whether they are satisfied with what they can achieve on a weight-loss programme – also predicts whether they will keep the weight off.

A survey in the magazine *Top Santé* points to what a serious problem body image is for women. The magazine reported that 95 per cent of those questioned were unhappy with their bodies, on a daily basis! We are told that 71 per cent said their body image was stopping them living the life they wanted; 64 per cent thought their whole life would be better if they were happy with their bodies; 46 per cent might change their career if they had a better body image; and 12 per cent might change a partner! Only 8 per cent said they were happy about their weight and only 7 per cent were happy about their shape. And do you know who was most likely to criticize their weight or shape? Other women.

Can we learn to love our bodies?

What can we do to make us kinder to each other and above all kinder to ourselves? Body dissatisfaction is now so common among girls and women of all ages (with or without eating disorders) that psychologists are beginning to wonder whether it should be classified as an illness. Asked to point to pictures that most closely resemble the shape and size of their body, women routinely pick women who are larger than themselves, a delusion also common among anorexics. However, Professor Glenn Waller, head of clinical psychology at St George's Hospital, London, told the Channel 4 health website that 85 to 90 per cent of women overestimate their size. He added, 'Can we still say that problems with body image are pathological if they affect nearly half the population?' Research carried out at Leeds University Medical School suggests that body image problems are often passed down through families. The research shows that from an early age children link being fat with being unintelligent, doing less well at school, being lazy and smelly and less liked by parents. In contrast, being skinny is associated with being successful and attractive and having lots of friends.

Programmes to improve body image and self-confidence with the goal of avoiding eating disorders – both overeating and anorexia – have been tried with children and adolescents in Australia and the USA, though not with great success. The approach is often to try and 'immunize' young people from the media images that promote the thin-ideal. Such efforts sometimes work in the short term, but the longer-term outcomes are far less encouraging. Long-term behavioural changes have been reported in only 3 out of 15 studies. And even though it may be possible to reduce young people's addiction to the thin-ideal, this doesn't automatically change their body dissatisfaction.

Some psychologists keep faith that attitudes and behaviour can be changed in a face-to-face situation. Lessons have been learned from the coping behaviour of some obese children, the more confident of whom seem to accept that they are as they are and that, anyway, it's not their fault. LighterLife counsellor Susan Murray works with people to improve self-esteem and body image as part of the programme to change attitudes to eating and exercise behaviour if you are to maintain weight loss:

You have to counter the belief that to be thin like Victoria Beckham is to be happy. It isn't that difficult because there's plenty of evidence that even if you are thin there is plenty of crap in your life. The trick is to find an alternative way of dealing with the crap rather than seeking refuge in food.

She gets clients to make lists of things they like about themselves as a start, and sets them small, achievable goals that they can pursue to improve how they look in order to encourage their self-confidence and body image.

Etre bien dans sa peau

There are some signs that this body loathing is culturally conditioned, Western and Northern European women being more vulnerable than those with Latin blood in their veins. It appears that Western attitudes to the thin-ideal are now infecting Asian women. But a comfortable plumpness still seems to find more favour round Eastern European, Mediterranean, Central and South American hips. Perhaps older peasant attitudes to female curves persist among these peoples.

Germaine Greer tells a story that illustrates how in some countries it is possible to believe that you are attractive even if you are not young, thin and beautiful. In a public loo in Sicily she saw a dumpy little middle-aged woman, with whiskers, a missing tooth and hair like a hedgehog, stand tip-toe to peer into the fly-blown mirror over the basin. '*Non sono bella; ma piacio,*' she said, with quiet satisfaction ('I'm not beautiful, but I'm attractive'). I bet *she* didn't want to be two kilos lighter.

7

Happy, healthy eating

An infinity of authors better qualified than I have written reams on the healthy diet, so I shall be brief. I will try to distinguish the 'happy, healthy diet' from the reducing diet, the self-denial diet or the fad diet. (See 'Don't be gulled by fad diets' on pp. 87–8.) Award-winning writer and broadcaster Leslie Kenton, author of more than 30 books on health, beauty and ageing, who generally talks a lot of sense, believes passionately that raw foods are superior to cooked. Cooking destroys some of the nutritional content of certain foods, so from this point of view her creed is justified by nutritional science. But there are other nutritionally valuable foods that the human gut simply can't handle in their raw state – pulses, potatoes, rice or anything containing unexploded starch, and of course meat. (In extremis, as in our prehistoric past, the human digestion can derive goodness from raw flesh, but years of eating cooked meat have led to a decline in the special digestive juices required to break down raw tissue.) And there are other useful foods that are quite digestible but when raw make the human gorge rise – personally, I feel that way about oysters – so it is probably wise not to be doctrinaire when it comes to composing a healthy diet.

You need two sources to work out a diet that will help you maintain a happy, healthy weight: expert advice on what is in food and what makes some foods more valuable and others more harmful, plus your own honest assessment of what foods you loathe, like or cannot live without and that fit into your lifestyle.

Consulting the experts

There is, if anything, even more hullabaloo about food than there is about obesity. Forests of newsprint are churned out daily, hours of hot-air-time expended, telling you that your body will seize up if you don't consume alfalfa or if it becomes polluted with dreaded *trans fats.* (There is something in the fuss about trans fats. We cover them on p. 83. There is also something in alfalfa, but you won't come to any harm without it.)

Two leading authorities on health and diet in the UK are the British Dietetic Association and the British Nutrition Foundation, and these are the source of the scientific information in this chapter unless otherwise stated. (See Useful addresses, p. 107, for contact details.)

The British Dietetic Association (BDA) advises a balanced diet by dividing food into five groups: two groups – fruit and vegetables, and bread, pulses and potatoes – that should be eaten generously; two others – dairy produce, and meat, fish or other alternative protein – in moderation; plus a fifth – foods that contain a lot of fat and sugar (we all know the guilty foods) – that should be eaten sparingly. When it comes to drink, they recommend unlimited water; moderate amounts of unsweetened fruit juice, tea and coffee (without sugar and with only low-fat milk); limited alcohol; plus commercial sweetened and/or fizzy drinks as a no-no – and always read the contents on the label. This is the sketchiest summary of food for health. For a more detailed list of essential nutrients plus World Health Organization recommendations, visit <http://www.dietand fitnessresources.co.uk/diet_nutrition/nutrientsguide.htm>.

The health benefits of the 'five pieces of fruit or vegetables a day' recommended by the British government have been particularly well documented. They contain *antioxidants*, chemicals which help to prevent cell damage, repair damaged cells, and appear to be protective against heart disease, serious eye disease and some cancers. These valuable antioxidants are also found in wine (see the box 'A pinch of salt and a sip of wine' on pp. 86–7), which is one reason why *moderate* alcohol consumption appears to be beneficial to health.

Balanced, but enjoyable

CREs probably learn these general principles before they are out of school uniform. They eat a lot of fruit, fresh cooked vegetables (especially green ones) and salads, making sure the dressing includes olive, walnut or hazelnut oil (see the box 'Good and bad fats' on pp. 82–3) and not too much salt (see the box 'A pinch of salt and a sip of wine', pp. 86–7). They eat wholemeal pasta, rice and bread – unless, that is, they hate wholemeal grains, in which case they eat their beloved French baguette, white Basmati rice or lasagne but they eat *less* of it than they would the wholemeal version. The same principle works for butter. Butter is a naughty saturated fat. These are mostly of animal origin: meat fat and dairy products are saturated fats (again, see the box 'Good and bad fats' on pp. 82–3). If you quite like low-fat spreads and can't tell whether your mushrooms have been tossed in margarine or butter, then the health-conscious eater abjures butter. But some would rather eat *a very little* butter than a bland, commercial gloop (the author's personal opinion), and as long as it is always used sparingly, preferably unsalted, the harm done is minimal.

The idea behind 'a little of what you like' is that no one should try to live on a diet they don't enjoy. Depriving yourself of something you love and forcing yourself to eat something – for example, a bran cereal that to you tastes like sawdust – makes a doctrinaire slimming diet impossible to live with. Your goal in aiming for a healthy, happy diet should be to eat things you enjoy, but if they come into the group of foods that are high in fat, sugar or salt, you should eat them *infrequently* and *in small portions*. These occasional 'treats' will probably be among the things you remove (temporarily) if you decide it is time to take off a few extra pounds.

Andrea, one of our CRE case histories at the beginning of Chapter 6, reports an interesting experience.

> I started watching what I ate in my late teens. I banned sausages, pies, pizza, chips – all the obviously naughty things. Fortunately I really like salad and fruit so it wasn't too difficult. To save argument I used to tell people that I just didn't like the naughty things. My friends got used to it and thought I was just fussy. And the funny thing was, I really did start to dislike those naughty foods. As I got older I found it quite difficult to sort out what I truthfully didn't like, and what I had *taught* myself to dislike. But I have finally managed to become more honest. I actually like a fruit pie when the raspberries are bubbling crimson through the pastry. I really love ice-cream, so nowadays I eat these things just occasionally. But I can honestly say I never want to eat chips or pasta ever again. I genuinely don't like them.

If you can achieve Andrea's eating pattern, which majors on foods you enjoy but that contain all the essential nutrients, and allows the flourish of small, infrequent naughty treats, you should be able to keep to it indefinitely. And that is the essence of a successful happy, healthy maintenance diet.

Good and bad fats

If you become obsessed with the idea that all fat is bad and try to cut it out of your diet completely you will not be healthy, and you may get very cold. National guidelines recommend that no more that 30 per cent of your daily intake should come from fat. If you are a CRE you are more likely to favour 25 per cent and will ensure that this is composed of the most nourishing, least suspect form of fat.

Fat is a necessary component in a healthy diet, but not all fats are equal. The saturated fats you find in dairy produce and meat, particularly red meat, contribute to a build-up of a particular form of soluble fat circulating in the blood called *low-density lipoproteins*, or LDL (*lipo* from the Greek for fat). They are also known as 'bad' cholesterol, because cholesterol is composed of both LDL and *high-density lipoproteins* (HDL) – or 'good' cholesterol.

Most vegetable oils and fish oils are *polyunsaturated fatty acids* or PUFAs. These are essential to normal health and growth because the human body cannot make them itself. For this reason they are sometimes known as 'essential' fatty acids, or EFAs. They have the same calorie content as saturated fats, but they lower the levels of bad LDL in the blood without affecting the good HDL. A high consumption of olive oil was a factor identified by the Seven Countries Study (see p. 34 in Chapter 3) thought to contribute to a lower incidence of heart disease in Mediterranean countries.

PUFAs or EFAs are further divided into two sub-groups depending on small differences in the way the molecule is made up. The two groups are called omega-6 and omega-3 (just to make life even more confusing, they are occasionally referred to as w-6 and w-3, or even N-6 and N-3). We mentioned omega PUFAs in Chapter 4 in connection with the protection they provide against atherosclerosis – popularly but mistakenly known as 'hardening' of the arteries. (The walls of the arteries are actually softened and broken down by the deposits of fat: *atheros* is the Greek for porridge.) Omega-3 is found in fish, cold-water sea-food and some grains and nuts: wheat germ, soybeans, flaxseed, pecans and walnuts. It reduces the risk of heart disease and may also protect against depression. Omega-6, found in sunflower and safflower oil, also reduces the risk of heart disease, but can contribute to allergies and inflammation. EFAs are explained with comprehensive clarity at the Fish Foundation website, <http://www.fish-foundation.org.uk/>.

There is a fourth type of fatty acid you need to know about, and these are bad guys. They are trans fats – saturated fats that occur naturally in the milk or flesh of ruminants (cows and sheep) or their products. But the kind the health experts are worried about because consumption is increasing are made from vegetable oils that have been chemically altered by industrial processing or by frying at very high temperatures, so that they become solid or semi-solid. They are a major ingredient of snack foods, fried foods and commercially baked products. Some snack foods can be up to 45 per cent trans fat, and because they raise bad LDL cholesterol and lower the good HDL they also increase the risk of coronary heart disease. In fact, gram for gram, they appear to do this even more than natural saturated fats, and so are potentially worse for our health. In the UK there is currently no requirement to label goods for trans fats, so check the packaging for '*hydrogenated*' or '*partially hydrogenated fats*' or vegetable oils; the further up the list they appear, the more trans fats the product is likely to contain. However, since in general trans fats are found in cakes, biscuits, pastry, pies, fried food, take-aways and hard margarine – not the sort of foods that form a major part of a healthy, calorie-controlled diet – hopefully you won't be eating much of them.

Modifying the happy maintenance diet

A few people may need to modify the healthy diet outlined above. Those still growing or trying to develop muscle, such as children, those who do a great deal of physical work, body-builders, dancers and pregnant women, will require a slightly different balance of nutrients. They will need a greater proportion of protein in the diet than those who are trying to stop growing. Increasing the amount of protein in the diet and reducing the carbohydrate is also one way to reduce weight, as we saw when considering the Atkins diet in Chapter 4, especially if you don't have a great deal to lose. However, a carb-less diet is definitely not a healthy diet, and the vast slabs of meat and dairy produce recommended by Atkins do not qualify either. Roughage provided by whole grains and vegetables is especially important when you reduce your daily calorie consumption because this can have the uncomfortable effect of slowing down your gut, to put it delicately.

Finding what works for you

If you want to lose weight and stay healthy, but are already eating a restrained and balanced diet, where do you do it? Each person needs to work out an individual solution, but here are a few suggestions:

- *Keep a food diary for a week.* Go through it and strike out those things that will reduce calories without unbalancing the diet. Top of the list will be any sugary or fatty treats – a gram of fat is nine calories compared to a gram of protein's four. It is probably wise to limit the booze. Only alcohol comes close to fat with seven calories per gram, and alcohol has a well-known tendency to undermine resolve. But don't be a kill-joy: one (or possibly two) glass(es) of wine with dinner can definitely be classed as health-giving. (See the box 'A pinch of salt and a sip of wine' on pp. 86–7.)
- *Get a chart of calories and nutrients.* Keeping a diary is not something you have to do every time you put on three or four pounds. You will eventually begin to recall what you have eaten with honesty and accuracy, though everyone underestimates what they are eating to begin with. It's the same with drinking or smoking; if someone says they drink three units a day it usually turns out to be five, and if they say they smoke 40, it's probably nearer 50. A revealing experiment involves taking overweight people into hospital (seriously overweight; they won't put you in hospital if you are 10 or 20 pounds overweight), and then feeding them *on what they say they have been eating.* Most of them lose weight. However, one thing you will need is a reliable reference book, or website, to check up on things. Just as most of us underestimate what we eat, so memory tends to reduce the calories food contains. And since you are concerned to make your eating healthy you also need a guide to what nutrients are in your food (see Further reading).

- *Be realistic in your goals.* Weight lost slowly is more likely to stay off than massive weight lost following starvation. The weight lost after fasting is partly the emptying of the gut but also dehydration. If you have an attack of food poisoning or a bad cold that stops you eating you may lose two to four pounds, depending on your size and previous diet. This goes straight back on when you start eating normally again. Aim to lose between one and two pounds a week, and don't weigh yourself every day; weight fluctuates even when you are dieting. Be realistic about your goal weight too; a pound of fat contains 3,500 calories, so to lose a pound a week you need to cut out 500 calories a day.

- *Watch your portion size.* Some CREs diet by reducing quantity but keeping the content of their diet the same – everything, that is, except the fruit and veg part. It's difficult to calculate but certainly keeps the diet varied.

- *Don't nibble.* It is said that the average housewife consumes untold calories by licking the cake mixture from her fingers, eating the left-over Marmite 'soldiers' on her children's plates and finishing off the piece of pie that is too small to put back in the fridge. What my family calls 'the fridge mice' can be kept off by covering everything in the fridge or larder in cling-film. Andrea said that when she had children she started to nibble left-overs, so she taught herself that it was never too late: if it got into her mouth, she spat it out into a paper hankie before she could swallow it. Not nice, but useful.

- *Cut down on dinner.* There is an old saw that goes 'Breakfast like a king; lunch like a prince and dine like a pauper.' It works for many. The logic behind it is that a good breakfast helps boost the metabolic rate at a time when it is naturally rising and will give you energy for the day; a reasonable lunch helps you over the natural dip in metabolism and general alertness that affects most people in the early afternoon, whereas calories taken in the evening, when most people's metabolic rate is starting to come down and they are less active, are more likely to be stored. Either way, a cup of low-calorie soup and some fruit at dinnertime is the reducing regime of a number of CREs I spoke to. Cutting down on dinner is less noticeable if you take up some new activity at that time of day: swimming, a reading group, amateur theatricals or digging an allotment.

- *Increase exercise.* This really comes into the next chapter, but it fits too well with finding other things to do at dinnertime not to mention it.
- *Join a slimming group.* This doesn't work for everyone. Martin, our boredom-diet case history at the beginning of Chapter 6, said that when he tried Weight Watchers they put him on a diet that included more than he was currently eating. He also found many of the other dieters so lacking in confidence and motivation that it depressed him. Others say that groups bring out the competitive spirit in them and they strive to impress with what they have lost each week, and that the trainers are a fund of useful tips and information. (See Useful addresses for slimming group contacts.)

A pinch of salt and a sip of wine

Salt and alcohol don't fit neatly into the food groups from which you assemble a healthy diet. Both are good taken in the right quantities, but bad if you take too much.

Salt (sodium chloride) is vital for all living creatures and is present in all our body tissues and fluids. Your body can't make it, and since some of it is lost through your skin when you perspire, or if you shed tears, it is important that you replace it in what you eat and drink. And, health apart, a little salt brings out the flavour in food, though too much can swamp it. But although the body has mechanisms to excrete salt that is surplus to requirements, there is a direct link between blood pressure and the amount of salt in the diet – less of the one lowers the other. In addition some people appear to have an unexplained sensitivity to salt which makes them exceptionally vulnerable, and since there is no easy test for salt sensitivity, the current medical advice is to eat as little as possible. So if you have a taste for salty food – Marmite, crisps, smoked fish or olives – you should avoid adding salt to dishes at table, though you don't have to leave it out of the cooking.

It's stating the obvious to remind you that excessive alcohol consumption is bad for your health and for weight, but these days we hear more and more stories about the benefits of *moderate* alcohol consumption. The national recommendation is two to three units of alcohol per day for women and three to four units for men, though it's also a good idea to have the occasional alcohol-free day. The health penalties of alcohol consumption are chiefly associated with binge drinking – considered to be five or more units in a session. The health benefits are associated with the moderate consumption of wine, particularly red wine; they include a lowered risk of heart disease, and there may also be some protection against colds. (The consumption of wine, along with fruit, vegetables and monounsaturate olive oil, is thought to account for the lower incidence of heart disease in Mediterranean countries first noted in the Seven Countries Study.) Wine appears to restore the level of antioxidants in the blood: those chemicals that keep the body's cells in good repair.

Good wine has well-documented life-enhancing qualities, but so has getting a little tiddly. How can you be sure it is the former rather than the latter that motivates your drinking? Ask yourself the following questions.

- Do you prefer one wine to another or one Scotch or beer to another?
- Would you go without rather than drink wine, beer or Scotch that was not to your taste?
- Do you try to match what you drink to what you are eating?
- Are there foods you feel just don't go with alcohol – boiled eggs, cereal?
- Do you mix more than two types of alcohol during the evening?
- Have you ever made do with the bottle of cherry brandy bought at Prague airport years ago, because there was nothing else in the cupboard?

If you answered 'no' to two or more of the first four questions and 'yes' to either of the last two you are probably not a discriminating drinker and should try and reform.

Don't be gulled by fad diets

The British Dietetic Association also provides useful advice on how *not* to go about dieting. 'There is no quick fix,' they warn. Beware diets that involve

- 'miracle' foods that 'burn off' fat: the 'burning of fat' is a colourful but meaningless image; fat is removed by the process of metabolism (being broken into its constituent parts) and converted into energy and waste products;

- bizarre quantities of only one food or type of food – for example, grapefruit, meat or cabbage soup – or specific combinations of food;
- rigid menus, times to eat or limited food choice;
- suggested rapid weight loss of more than two pounds (one kilogram) a week;
- failing to warn people who suffer from diabetes, high blood pressure or kidney disorder that they should seek medical advice before slimming;
- focusing on appearance rather than health.

The BDA is pretty ruthless on the concept of the 'detox diet' too. The idea that the body needs to be 'cleansed', cleared of 'toxic waste', especially after a period of excess like Christmas, is, it explains, a myth.

> Our body constantly filters out, breaks down and excretes toxins and waste products. These could include alcohol, medications, products of metabolism and digestion, dead cells, chemicals from pollution and bacteria. This is achieved by our in-built 'detoxifiers' – the liver, the kidneys, skin, intestines and lungs. If we generally follow a healthy diet and lifestyle, they work in harmony to do the job rather well and we don't need special help.

Supplementary paragraph

The BDA also talks sense on supplements. If you eat a balanced diet you probably don't need supplements, with four notable exceptions: folic acid (400 micrograms a day) if you are pregnant; calcium and vitamin D if you are at risk of osteoporosis (the thinning of bone that particularly affects women after the menopause); a vitamin D supplement for breast-feeding women and infants under two years old; a supplement of vitamin B12 for strict vegans (most of us get this from meat or dairy products).

These groups apart, the BDA says, if you want to take supplements 'as an insurance policy choose a general multi-vitamin/mineral supplement that provides at least 15 nutrients at levels at or below 150 per cent of the EC Recommended Daily Amount'. And this should be marked on the packaging.

This is only a whistle-stop tour of happy, healthy eating. If you feel the need of more detailed advice, follow up some of the sources recommended at the back of the book, but remember, eating should be enjoyable and whenever possible sociable and it won't be if you make too much of a performance about it. It is, after all, only part of a happy, healthy life.

8

Long live exercise

I have to declare an interest – as they say in government circles – when it comes to exercise. Whatever the scientific evidence, and the same hyped-up claims and assumptions bedevil this field as confuse the dossier on overweight and health, my personal experience of taking regular exercise somewhat late in life has been beneficial: for my weight and health, but particularly for my well-being. As it happens my position is supported by leading health and exercise expert Steven Blair of the Cooper Institute in Texas. Activity may not be the secret of life for everyone, he concedes; human beings vary in every trait that anyone has measured, so they probably vary in the health benefit they gain from identical doses of exercise. But to return to Blair's assessment:

> In the absence of definitive evidence of how big this benefit (from exercise) is I support the statement of the American College of Sports Medicine (ACSM) and the US Centers for Disease Control and Prevention (CDC) that people who do at least moderate amounts of activity seem to be a whole lot better off as a group.

Let's look at *how* better off in more detail.

Why should physical activity be important for health?

We hear it said so often it is easily taken for granted. The evolutionary argument goes something like this: in his primitive state *Homo sapiens* depended for survival on chasing his prey and running away from those that wished to prey upon him. Hence the human body evolved as an organism adapted to physical activity, not to sitting on a sofa opposite a screen with moving pictures. A similar line of thought promotes the importance of roughage and the inappropriateness of refined flour or sugar in the diet. In our primitive and rural state carbohydrates were husky whole grains; meat protein was hard to catch, cook and prepare; sugar was only available at low levels in fruit or small quantities in natural honey – hence high-fat sugary processed foods with the fibre taken out are all wrong for our bodies.

The seventeenth-century English poet John Dryden voiced the modern view.

> Better to hunt in fields, for health unbought,
> Than fee the doctor for a nauseous draught.
> The wise, for cure, on exercise depend;
> God never made his work, for man to mend.
> (Epistle: 'To my honoured kinsman John Driden' (1700) 1.92)

These are persuasive ideas but not exactly scientific evidence. We can't compare the health of primitive man with the modern couch-potato, and if we could we would probably find that our ancestor was riddled with parasites and died before he had time to develop the conditions that afflict the couch-potato anyway. But we can compare contemporaries who are active and those who are not. And there is clear evidence that activity – and put aside for one moment how much or what kind, or whether it actually affects what you weigh – makes people both healthier and happier.

It's worth remembering that the fitness that follows physical exercise will not necessarily make you slim. It could make you heavier, because muscle weighs more than fat. There are any number of Hollywood stars with muscles honed in the gym who, on the basis of their BMI, would be classified as overweight: Brad Pitt and Mel Gibson, for example. And Russell Crowe and George Clooney on the same scale would be rated obese.

Fit does not mean slim

At the Cooper Institute's Aerobics Center longitudinal study, Blair and his colleagues have tracked the health, weight and basic fitness levels of more than 70,000 people over more than twenty years. Unlike many studies, they do not depend on self-report – dangerously inaccurate as seen. The Aerobics Center regularly calls in those in the study to do treadmill stress tests, which enable them to record pulse rate (and the time it takes to return to normal after exercise), heart rate, respiration rate and maximum intake of oxygen – standard measures of fitness. They then relate these to the participant's weight and body mass. They have discovered that weight and body mass have no relevance whatsoever to health and fitness. Even people with a BMI of 30 or higher who engage in only moderate levels of physical activity have half the mortality rates of sedentary people who maintain a supposedly 'ideal' weight. This remains true even if the weight is contributed by fat, rather than muscle. Overall, the health and mortality of the heavy, active people are identical to those of the active, 'ideal'-weight people. Activity is the key.

Exercise when?

This is an interesting finding that will comfort those of us who only started to take health seriously when we turned 40. There is evidence that being active during your youth does not contribute as much to health as exercise or moderate activity in middle age – though this should not be taken as the OK for children and teenagers to stay in bed or in front of a screen all day, abandoning exercise. The Harvard Alumni Study has followed one-time Harvard students since 1988. They are divided into three categories: athletes; those who did sport for more than five hours a week, and those who did sport for less than five hours a week; there was no category for couch-potatoes. Assessed in middle age, it turns out that there is no difference in terms of cardiovascular health in those who had continued to be physically active all their lives, those who had been active as students but let it all drop once they left college, and those who only took up physical activity in later life.

Reduced cardiovascular risk is the health benefit most often put forward as the major benefit of regular activity, so it is surprising to find that all the Harvard sports jocks derived no advantage from a lifetime of pretty dedicated activity. But other researchers have found the same phenomenon. In their chapter in *Perspectives on Health and Exercise*, Boreham and Riddoch say, 'Although we feel instinctively that physical activity ought to be beneficial to the health of children, there is surprisingly little empirical evidence to support this notion.' The authors say that although there is evidence that exercise improves blood pressure and general fitness, as measured by the Cooper Institute's longitudinal study, it remains to be demonstrated whether this also leads to a longer lifetime or better health.

Many health benefits are claimed for exercise, but only a few are at all robust when it comes to the young. From another Harvard Alumni study we find that physical activity in youth may reduce the incidence of stroke in middle-aged men, and from yet other studies that it may lower the risk of colon cancer and breast cancer. However, you have to take into account the fact that strenuous sporting activity (Harvard athletes) in itself carries a health risk; sporting injuries are responsible for secondary osteoarthritis – the kind that results from damaged joints as opposed to wear and tear over a lifetime – and worse. In fact, Gard and Wright, quoting another group of researchers, say,

> On a purely cost–benefit basis they advocate sedentary living for young people and moderate physical activity among the middle-aged and elderly because the health care costs incurred by young people as a result of exercising outweigh the long term health care saving of this physical activity.

The problem with measuring health benefit in the young, as we discovered when assessing the percentage of 'extra premature deaths' (see Chapter 3), is that in the Western world most of the young are pretty healthy and very few (at most 20 per cent) die at that age, so that the mortality and morbidity rates within which different groups may experience different degrees of risk are small.

It's different when we come to middle and old age. For this age group even arch sceptics Gard and Wright acknowledge that physical activity is of value, though they say that there is a lack of firm evidence as to how much or of what sort. On the assumption that you get the quantity and quality right, you can reasonably expect not only improved fitness – as measured by the Cooper Institute longitudinal study – but more energy, greater strength and flexibility, less lower-back pain and even improved sleep and general well-being, though this is more difficult to measure. On the health side, you should be at reduced risk of the following age-related conditions:

- heart attack (risk reduced with as little as 150 calories physical activity a day – approximately a brisk mile walk);
- stroke (reduced by 20–40 per cent);
- type 2 diabetes (reduced by 30 per cent);

- hip fracture (reduced by 40 per cent);
- colon cancer (reduced by 10–46 per cent).

Exercise how?

Those of you who were exercise-conscious in the 1980s will remember the Jane Fonda workout: the urge to 'feel the burn', not to mention the tights and leggings that made us look like refugees from the ballet school. At this time people were urged to do an hour or more a day pumping iron at the gym to get that 'perfectly toned' body.

But in recent years the amount of physical activity recommended for health has been revised downwards: what Americans call 'exercise lite'. For a moment put to one side whether the physical activity required to maintain health in middle age will also reduce your weight – quite likely not. The reason for the revision was that researchers discovered that most estimates of how much activity people were having depended on self-report, and whereas it was pretty easy for them to recall how often and how long they had been at the gym or had gone swimming or salsa dancing, it was much more difficult for them to keep a record of how much gardening, running to catch a bus, or pounding up and down stairs they had done, so that the contribution of routine daily activity tended to be underestimated in research studies. People are now usually asked to estimate how 'sedentary' they are over the average day – for example, do they sit at a desk from nine in the morning until six at night? If you do, then the usual recommendation is that you require more formally organized physical activity than, say, the mother of three children under ten who lives in a top-floor flat and goes about on foot or by public transport.

The other reason that the recommended level of physical activity was scaled down is that most research is done on young, relatively healthy populations (college students are the most researched group in the Western world). The young need to do significantly more exercise to have a measurable effect on health risk factors like body fat, blood pressure and cholesterol levels, and tend to start from a baseline of higher routine daily and night-time activity than the middle-aged and elderly. Research suggests that among the elderly, already unhealthy and less fit, a significant health bonus can be achieved by even modest increases in physical activity. Such people don't need to be sweating it out at the gym for an hour every day. Just taking the stairs and walking the dog may be beneficial. National guidelines in the UK and the USA recommend 30 minutes of moderate-intensity physical activity at least five and preferably seven days a week, this level of activity being defined as walking at about three to four miles an hour – that's a brisk walk. Anyone over 45 not already taking regular, formal exercise should aim for this level.

To decide whether this will be adequate, start by making an estimate of what your routine daily physical activity involves: how often do you walk briskly or run, climb stairs, garden, do DIY, dance? If you reckon that this is less than two and a half hours a week, or even about that, top it up with something more formal. After all, the cut-off point for the bottom-of-the-activity-ladder group in the Harvard Alumni study was twice that – five *hours* a week.

At this level you should start to be fitter and healthier, provided it is an advance on what you were doing before. But unless it is combined with a considerable reduction in calories, you may not actually lose weight. To do this you will probably need to do even more, or something slightly different.

Exercise for people who can't hit balls

When embarking on increased physical activity it's really important to do something you enjoy, otherwise boredom, strain or competition from more attractive alternative activities may make you give up. It was easy enough when you were young. Eight-year-olds can run after a ball or a dog for hours on end without becoming breathless or being aware of any effort. Teenagers hump their sports gear out every weekend and happily get covered in mud and glory on the pitch. Even in our twenties we jived, bopped or otherwise danced the night away for the fun of meeting the opposite sex and hearing the latest music. If you have small children, just keeping up with them and avoiding making a fool of yourself in the Parents' Race is incentive enough for a fair amount of physical activity.

The real challenge is when you hit middle and old age. The shadow of the rocking chair haunts us all. Even though nowadays grannies are as likely to be jogging in a tracksuit as knitting with a shawl round their shoulders, vigorous activity doesn't come naturally to the middle-aged; it requires deliberate effort. Though of course there is always golf. If you have an eye for a ball there are physical activities aplenty to gee up your metabolic rate. But if hitting balls is not your thing, or if the ball was a snooker ball played in a smoke-filled billiard hall, you need to be more inventive.

Emma says

Even at school I hated sport. It was the clothes, the smell of gym-shoes, and the awful people. I was a spindly, four-eyed swot, the one always picked last for the team. I couldn't wait to give up chasing balls. Then, after my children were born, I put on some weight. I was active, but I suppose I was snacking more. I always seemed to be in the kitchen. I joined a group with the idea of losing a few pounds and met Jocelyn. She suggested we went salsa dancing. It was a wow. We had such fun it didn't even feel like exercise. I'm sure it's the chief reason I got back into shape. Now I sometimes go twice a week and manage to fit in yoga as well and I feel a lot fitter. It's not about weight any more, it's about enjoying life.

Edna says

I was getting low and generally lethargic and had bouts of severe depression. I was spending more and more time in the doctor's waiting room. And then my daughter showed me a photo of us all swimming when she was young. 'You were a great swimmer you know, Mum. Do you think you could teach the grandchildren?' It was a revelation. I now take them swimming at the weekend or on a summer evening, but I also go for myself. Every day either I walk or I go for a swim. The difference it has made to my physical and mental health is amazing.

Jo says

One of my mates got me to take on an allotment. I didn't think I'd have the energy. I'd been spending too much time in bed or in front of the telly since I retired, but now I'm down there all weathers. The beans and the spinach and potatoes are coming along fine; it really gives you a lift to grow your own veg. And I've made a whole new load of friends.

Chris and Vicky say

When we were young we went on walking holidays, but as we got older Vicky's knees began to play up and we walked less and less. And the less she walked the worse the joints became, and I know I was putting on the pounds. But then our son gave us this Labrador puppy.

We just had to take her out to burn off the energy, otherwise she would tear the furniture to pieces. I thought Vicky wouldn't be able to make it. But she comes along, and the joints are not as stiff now she is getting some exercise again.

Case histories like these demonstrate that activity doesn't have to be exercise and exercise does not mean becoming an athlete. The secret is either to find something you enjoy that just incidentally includes physical activity or, alternatively, find something to do *while* you exercise. This is why you see the joggers in the park with music plugged into their ears and why the exercise bike in the gym comes equipped with a mini-screen showing you a choice of videos. Andrea does cardiovascular exercise in the form of pounding up and down the two flights of stairs in her Victorian house for 15 to 30 minutes every day. When she started, she says, she had to count to make sure she was doing the right number of runs; now, she is so used to it she runs up and down the required number of times automatically and she can listen to her portable radio or even read a magazine while she does it – being careful not to bump into one of the children as she goes.

If you decide to do formal exercise for the first time in middle age, it pays to consult an expert first, and your doctor if you are in any doubt about your general health. A good gym will have a physiotherapist or experienced trainer to assess your age and fitness and advise you as to what level of intensity to start at. Whether you exercise under professional guidance or alone, it pays to follow a carefully graduated programme. Some current useful books and websites are listed in Further reading.

There are three parts to an exercise programme. The first is warming up – stretching, bending, twisting and generally getting your muscles warm and loosened up before putting demands on them. This is followed by *aerobic exercise* – exercise that taxes the body, and particularly the cardiovascular system. It should be of reasonable duration – between 15 and 60 minutes – and you should feel your heart rate and pulse speeding up as your body uses oxygen to convert the glucose in your blood into energy. This cardiovascular exercise is what conditions the heart and lungs and gradually increases your endurance. You will probably be breathless and begin to sweat. The third part of an exercise programme is winding down, while your blood pressure, pulse and heart rate return to normal.

'Resistance is useful'
(With acknowledgement to the *Guardian* newspaper.)

Under this headline the *Guardian* ran an article on some ongoing research at Glasgow University of particular interest to those who want to use exercise for weight control as well as for fitness and health. According to researcher Dr Niall MacFarlane, the rate at which fat is burned during exercise can be increased as much as threefold by doing what is called *resistance training* for 20 minutes prior to aerobic exercise.

Resistance training is really a form of weightlifting, using mainly the weight of your own body to increase the load you put on your muscles and cardiovascular system. Unlike exercise that involves elevation – jumping or jogging – resistance exercise does not shock the load-bearing joints, which can be a problem for middle-aged exercisers. The most familiar resistance exercises are push-ups, sit-ups, squats and lunges, but you could also lift light weights. MacFarlane explains his use of the popular term 'burn fat'. It doesn't involve smoke, flames or melting, it involves fat-oxidation – using oxygen to break down fat. 'Resistance training helps switch on the body's fat-oxidation processes quicker. It also means people will be able to endure longer subsequent aerobic exercise.' The reason people are usually told to exercise for at least half an hour is that at the start of a session the body fuels the energy expended with sugars or carbohydrates stored in muscle and the liver; this can lead to fatigue, so that they often give up before their body moves from burning up carbohydrate to burning up the energy stored in fat. The Glasgow team believes that 20 minutes of resistance enables the body to access fat as an energy source sooner. If they are right, you might be able to reduce exercise time to an hour three times a week. The fat-burning potential of 20 minutes' resistance plus 40 minutes' aerobic exercise – say, brisk walking – would be the equivalent of two hours' aerobic-only exercise.

Try it: it may work; and watch for further reports from Glasgow. At the time of writing, the team had only worked with 11 fit volunteers. If they can confirm their results with several thousand unfit 50-year-olds, they are definitely in business.

Effect of exercise on mood and psyche

Exercise and activity do not just act on the body; they have a measurable effect on mood. Exercise leads to the release of a number of naturally occurring chemicals that have an effect on the brain. The *endorphins*, or natural painkillers, released by the body when it is in pain or under stress, have a similar effect to a group of powerful pain-killing drugs called *opiates*, which include morphine and heroin. The reason these drugs can lead to abuse is that they produce a wonderful feeling of euphoria. An equivalent but less extreme sensation is experienced by people who exercise: 'the runner's high', said to be experienced by 60–70 per cent of well-conditioned runners.

Endorphins have been found to increase to as much as five times their resting levels during a prolonged bout of aerobic exercise (more than 30 minutes). This varies from person to person and is affected by how much regular exercise or sporting activity they do. The body develops tolerance to opiate drugs, and something similar happens with the endorphins released following exercise. The more regularly you exercise, the more you need to do to get the same high. So, as with opiate drugs, exercise can become addictive, leading some athletes to give up other activities in pursuit of the ever-receding endorphin 'fix'. This is probably not a problem for most of us, but be warned if you have a tendency towards addiction of any sort.

Exercise also has an effect on important neurotransmitters – chemical messengers – in the brain. It increases the level of serotonin, and depletion of serotonin in the brain is associated with depression. So exercise can give you a lift as well as a high.

Fiona's story

Fiona was struck down with depression after the birth of her second child. She had also put on some weight, and her doctor suggested she undertake a fitness programme that included modifications to her diet and regular exercise. It worked. 'I began to realize that exercising was the only time I felt the fog lift. After a workout I felt energized, revived. I felt human again. I remember telling my husband and my mum, "Make me go to the gym. I have to go." Sometimes I think my workouts were the only things holding me together.'

There are other, less easily measured psychological benefits from exercise. A number of studies of those taking regular vigorous exercise of various sorts – dancing as well as conventional exercise routines – have identified something called the Mastery Hypothesis: this suggests that exercise enhances mood because it triggers a sense of achievement. Mastering a new skill or practising an established one makes us feel accomplished, capable, competent, and may well also have a positive effect on mood. There is another theory, the Distraction Hypothesis, which suggests that exercise alleviates depression by temporarily distracting us from the everyday stresses of our lives, and yet another that suggests that it is the social interaction of many of these activities – playing games, dancing, walking with the dog – that lifts the mood.

The concept of 'mastery' chimes with what the CREs say, and with the experience of the CBT counsellors with LighterLife. If you can boost your confidence and self-esteem, and take charge of your life, you can become fitter, lose weight, do anything. The world is your oyster.

Much remains uncertain in these ideas. If they do exist, do they affect everyone, or just some, or all of us but variably? Can we learn these behaviours? Can attitudes be learned or are they a question of your individual personality?

One word of warning. You can do all these things and still get ill. Exercise may be protective against many things but it can't make you live for ever, and even the fit, the happy and the healthy are struck down, through no fault of their own. It is said that as Jackie Onassis was dying of cancer at the age of 64 she complained bitterly of the sacrifices she had made to stay fit. 'Why did I do all those push-ups?' Paul Campos reminds us that the fitness cult may be driven by 'a subconscious belief that people who die have committed some basic error in their workout routine, and/or have eaten one too many Twinkies'.

Dying or getting ill is not a sin. You are not being punished, nor are you a failure if you do not remain for ever healthy, fit or slim. Some things are in our stars, or at any rate in our genes. This is something we look at in the last chapter.

9

'What must I do to be saved?'

This book started by looking at how the idea of being fat or over-weight became linked in the popular imagination, not just with beauty, but with health and even with sin. This last chapter returns to this theme because when you start to consider the life-goals people set themselves you realize that they are personal, emotional, possibly socially or religiously conditioned, but are rarely rational or scientific.

We live in an age and a society that respects the laws of evidence, and science is held to offer tested evidence and to be the basis of known fact. We no longer consult chicken entrails or tea-leaves for guidance – although the persistence of belief in the influence of the stars on our personalities and destinies reveals that belief is not always conditional on the most exigent standards of evidence – but because most of us have only a limited understanding of science we consult experts about what it proves. They are our equivalent of read-ing the runes, consulting the Oracle or the Holy Book. But the insub-stantial nature of our trust is exposed when science comes up against older, established faith, as in Creationism versus Darwin's theory of evolution. This particular debate reveals how selective most people are when it comes to evidence. They welcome the evidence that supports their belief or point of view, but they don't want to be confused by anything that challenges it.

In my view, that is what has happened to the issue of being over-weight. Science has been recruited to support a point of view: that obesity is unhealthy, not to say slothful or even sinful; and the evidence that questions this view has been dismissed as 'giving people permission to be fat'. We have to ask ourselves: do we want to be a certain 'ideal' weight *because* science says it will make us healthy and long-lived, or do we want to be that weight and then gather scientific evidence to justify it?

I think we should go further in questioning our pursuit of an ideal weight and even of ideal health. Are these the right questions to be asking science to answer for us? Science is at its best when we can do controlled experiments that answer questions like: if I do this, then what? Or, what is this made of? It gets closest to answering questions about how living systems work when we look at animals, preferably small ones like fruit flies that reproduce at a rate of knots, because at least with animals you can compare one intervention with another and say with confidence that doing this seems to demonstrate this or that result in a certain number of cases. But studying living systems is not like physics; even with animals you rarely get an answer that tells you what will happen in 100 per cent of cases. And with human beings we don't do truly controlled experiments – it wouldn't be ethical – so the percentages become smaller and the sub-groups affected or not affected become more numerous. It's a bit like comparing humans with chimpanzees: 98 per cent of their genetic code may be the same but the detail is in the difference. Human beings are in many obvious ways alike, but in infinitely subtle, important ways different.

It's a puzzlement. And yet it is the doctor's role to do something about things, even when knowledge is at best partial. When something has clearly gone wrong – the patient has a fever, a broken leg, cannot keep food down – there are scientifically validated ways to put things right, or at very least to improve matters or make the patient more comfortable while he or she recovers or dies. But ask doctors about achieving health and their feet shuffle; their eyes shift. Prescriptions for health, though clearly highly desirable, are elusive. Safer perhaps to define the thing that is to be treated as an illness. Hence the obesity epidemic.

Gard and Wright, in the course of *The Obesity Epidemic*, their scholarly rebuttal of vast swathes of obesity research, challenge the idea of treating the body as a machine. It is not like a machine; each one is different and the systems that compose it work in a mysterious way their wonders to perform. Since the body is not a machine, it is small wonder, they say, that we get so few definitive answers about why some are one weight and some another, and about what connection there is between health and weight. At the end of the book, they have this to say:

> Science is an important element in our lives but it is not the source of all truths and the fact that people do not think as scientifically

as scientists is, on balance, a good thing. In the case of obesity science, scientists themselves do not think as scientifically as they might imagine themselves to do. The trouble is many scientists will interpret this point as a criticism when, in fact, the ability to think beyond science is a great untapped resource.

It is attractive to class some phenomenon as an illness because then we are justified in calling on medical science to correct it. And of course, those who supply the corrective treatment can make a lot of money. Science can improve our mood, help us cope with the change of life, sort out children who are hyperactive and inattentive, and possibly even improve our memory, but that doesn't mean these human experiences are illnesses. Being healthy, being happy, being vigorous and alert despite old age are better viewed as life-goals.

Changing life-goals and how to achieve them

I expect you have picked up this book because you would like to be healthy and you believe that what you weigh may have something to do with it. Health is a life-goal that came into fashion in the early years of the twentieth century and has endured into the twenty-first. It emerged partly because at that time advances in public health suddenly increased people's chances of staying alive. Before that, simply surviving infancy – in some Western European countries up to 350 children per 1,000 live births died – surviving childbirth if you were a woman, and reaching your full three-score years and ten was an exceptional achievement; life expectancy was between 35 and 40 years. Health is still a luxury beyond achievable life-goals for people born in Africa.

To some extent, whether you believe you are healthy or not depends on testable evidence. You can safely say that you are not healthy if you have a condition that modern medicine can remedy. There are in fact fewer conditions like this than you might think. Modern medicine vaccinates or inoculates against childhood ailments, cures infections, corrects deficiencies and repairs damage with amazing skill. But with many conditions, and in particular the disease of middle age, it can only offer treatment. Other more complicated, less easily treatable conditions are not even universally regarded as illness (or non-health): spots, headaches, colds and aches and pains, failing memory, depression. Some people believe that things that are either disabling or disruptive of life should also be remedied by medicine, whereas others just accept them as part of being a vulnerable human being. Being overweight or obese comes into this category. It is not illness, though in extremes it may add to health risk and/or become disabling.

Humans are ambitious creatures; we have so many life-goals to choose from. The life-goals of 'life, liberty and the pursuit of happiness' are written into the US constitution, and we are now seeing the rise of 'Happiness Studies'. We don't have a constitution in the UK; nevertheless, in my own lifetime I have seen a panorama of different life-goals rise and fade away. The post-war generation in which I grew up adopted the goal of Voltaire's Candide – *'cultiver son jardin'* – to put their own little patch in order because the world had just been turned upside down by the Second World War. The Sixties flower-children, reared on free milk, health and state education, espoused the goals of 'peace and love' and 'make love not war', and experimented with 'the Good Life' of self-sufficiency or life on a commune. I have seen the emergence of the 'me-generation', ruled by the Thatcherite principle that 'greed is good' or the L'Oréal one that you should have it 'because you're worth it', and finally I have seen a generation emerge that believes the goal of the good life is not fouling our own nests or destroying our planet.

Goodness and happiness are elusive commodities. We are lucky to be secure enough to seek for them. You can't legislate for them – though governments have tried – and you can't test for them, although social scientists have attempted to measure life-satisfaction. They found that it depended on having a job or role in life that you enjoyed, where you felt valued and where you were not pushed around. It depended on a rich network of friends and family, on feeling secure and on being active and learning new things all your life, and that it depended on not feeling a lot worse off than the next person. A recent study from the British Medical Association reported a steady increase in mental health problems among children between 5 and 16 years old. Nearly 10 per cent suffer from psychological problems that are 'persistent, severe and affect functioning on a day-to-day basis'. Roughly 1.1 million children under the age of 18 'would benefit from specialist services'. In the media hands were held up in horror: a childhood depression epidemic! It occurred to me that possibly, if they had done such surveys in the nineteenth century, they would have discovered that children who had to go down mines, up chimneys or work 16 hours with dangerous factory machinery were depressed. Or perhaps not. Since this was the lot of all children like them, perhaps they just accepted it as the way things were.

Because, of course, this is the problem about having goals, like those wonderful 'choices' the government always promises us. Goals have to be achievable. If you can't achieve them – like being on the front cover of *Vogue*, winning the lottery or playing for Man United – they only make you dissatisfied with yourself.

Settling for the possible

In the days before mass communications it was possible for the 'poor man at the gate' to have little idea of what it was like to be the 'rich man in his castle' and consequently not to envy him. These days we dine out on a diet of celebrity lifestyles in the pages of *Now* and *Hello!* which encourage us to dream of impossible levels of wealth, fitness, fame and success. Wise diet counsellors set achievable goals that will boost confidence and improve body image and make their clients feel 'good in their skin'. Reaching for goals within your grasp is empowering.

You want to be healthy and a healthy weight. Health, like happiness, can be elusive. Sometimes it's easier to find it by forgetting it for a moment. If your life-goals encourage you to be self-obsessed it won't help you to be either. Look up from the scales and away from the mirror. What's going on outside the window? Go out and get involved. Lose yourself in something that really absorbs you: dancing, making music, learning a new language, cultivating your garden. Do things *with* other people and *for* other people, because there is nothing like giving to others to make you feel richer. If you don't have any young children around, see if you can find some; doing things with young children, or young animals and young plants for that matter, is invigorating. It may not make you live for ever but it will make the life you do have a great deal more enjoyable. Don't take my advice; work it out for yourself. You don't need science to discover what makes you happy. You're the expert on that. Go out and do it and your health and your weight can look after themselves.

Useful addresses

Nutrition, weight and fitness support and information

British Dietetic Association
5th Floor, Charles House
148/9 Great Charles Street
Queensway
Birmingham B3 3HT
Tel.: 0121 200 8080
Website: www.bda.uk.com/weightwise.html

British Nutrition Foundation
High Holborn House
52–54 High Holborn
London WC1V 6RQ
Tel.: 020 7404 6504 (multiple lines)
Website: www.nutrition.org.uk
Email: postbox@nutrition.org.uk

Keep Fit Association
Astra House
Suite 1.05
Arklow Road
London SE14 6EB
Tel.: 020 8692 9566
Website: www.keepfit.org.uk
Email: kfa@keepfit.org.uk

LighterLife UK Ltd
Cavendish House
Parkway
Harlow Business Park
Harlow
Essex CM19 5QF
Tel.: 08700 664747
Website: www.lighterlife.com
Email: inform@lighterlife.com

Overeaters Anonymous (Great Britain)
PO Box 19
Stretford
Manchester
M32 9EB
Helpline: 07000 784985 (numbers and meetings throughout UK)
Website: www.oagb.org.uk
(Website includes details of Overeaters Anonymous around the world)

Pilates Foundation UK Limited
PO Box 57060
London EC4P 4XB
Tel.: 07071 781859
Website: www.pilatesfoundation.com/contacts.php
(Website provides details of local Pilates studios)

Weight Watchers UK
Customer Services Direct Line: 0845 345 1500
Class Enquiries Line: 0845 7 123 000
Website: www.weightwatchers.co.uk

Useful websites

www.ashwell.uk.com/shape.htm
The Ashwell Shape Chart.

**www.channel4.com/health/microsites/0-9/4health/food/
abe_image.html**
Contains an article, 'How can we learn to love our bodies?', by Jenny Bryan,
on body image in general.

**www.dietandfitnessresources.co.uk/diet_nutrition/nutrientsguide.
html**
Provides nutrition information.

www.fish-foundation.org.uk
Explains the role in nutrition and health of omega-3 polyunsaturates from
fish and fish oils.

www.fitnwell.net/Your%20BMI.htm
An easily viewed site for BMI tables showing underweight, overweight and
obesity bands.

www.halls.md
Extremely erudite US site covering all areas of weight and health, BMI tables
and Met Life tables. Check your BMI; check it against what your age-group
would like to be. Reasoned criticism and endless references.

www.thehistoryof.net/the-history-of-dieting.html
A self-explanatory site from Vancouver.

www.ukwellness.com/
The broadly helpful website of UKWellness, which provides information
and contacts for a range of medical conditions plus exercise, lifestyle, fitness
and weight loss.

www.wlsinfo.org.uk
Provides details of weight loss surgery.

Appendix: body-mass index (BMI) chart

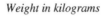

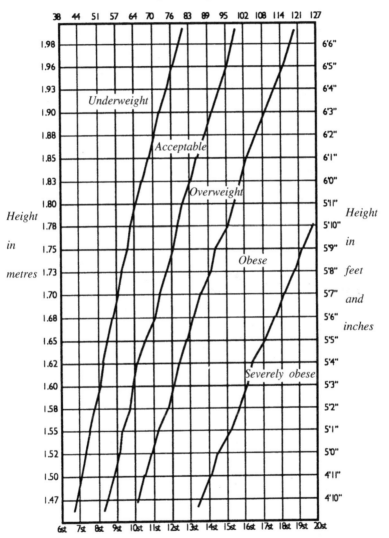

Weight in kilograms

Weight in stones

Glossary

Aerobic exercise muscular activity that conditions the heart and lungs by increasing the efficiency with which the body uses oxygen to convert glucose in the blood into energy.

Android 'man'-shaped or boyish.

Antioxidants chemicals found in some foods that neutralize free radicals and prevent them from damaging DNA.

Arteriosclerosis hardening of the arteries due to deposits of calcium in the walls, mostly due to ageing; different from atherosclerosis (see below).

Arthritis inflammation of the joints.

Atheroma a build-up of fatty deposits on the lining of arteries, increasing the risk of heart disease or stroke.

Atherosclerosis narrowing of the arteries due to deposits of fats (see cholesterol) in the vessel walls, which roughen their surface allowing clots to form on them, increasing the risk of heart attack, stroke, and kidney and eye problems.

Bioelectrical impedance analysis passing a low-level current through the body to calculate the proportion of fatty tissue, which impedes the passage of the current, compared with muscle, through which it passes more easily.

Carbohydrate one of the three main nutrient groups in food, derived principally from sugars and starches like potatoes and cereals. The other groups are proteins and fats.

Cardiovascular relating to the heart and blood vessels (arteries, veins and capillaries); the circulation.

Cholesterol a substance made by the body and derived primarily from animal fat, which may be increased by a high-fat diet, leading to a build-up of fatty plaques in blood vessels and increasing the risk of heart disease and stroke. (See high-density and low-density lipoproteins.)

Cognitive behaviour therapy a psychological technique aimed at converting negative thought patterns and attitudes into positive and constructive ones.

Congestive heart failure weakness of the heart muscle which results in it failing to pump all the blood from the heart. The back-up in the blood vessels causes a build-up of fluid in body tissues.

Coronary artery or heart disease a build-up of fatty material in the wall of the coronary arteries (atheroma) that causes narrowing of the vessels, restricting the flow of blood and thus of oxygen to the heart. Oxygen starvation of the heart muscle can lead to a heart attack.

Diabetes an incurable disease signalled by elevated levels of sugar in the blood; caused either by the failure of the pancreas to produce insulin, or by the development of resistance to the action of normal amounts of insulin produced by the pancreas, or both.

DNA (deoxyribonucleic acid) the chemical building blocks inside the nucleus of cells that carry genetic information – the mechanism by which heredity works.

Endorphins hormone-like chemicals that act in the brain to block pain and promote a positive mood.

Epidemiological studies studies that relate the incidence, distribution and possible causes of disease within and between populations.

Gastric banding or by-pass the insertion, by surgery, of a sleeve or band round the stomach to narrow it and reduce its capacity, or a tube to by-pass it completely.

Gastro-oesophageal reflux disease (GORD) regurgitation of digestive juices from the stomach into the oesophagus which sometimes reach the mouth.

Glycaemic index a way of measuring the speed with which a particular type of food is broken down and converted into blood-sugar (glucose).

Glycogen the form in which blood-sugar (glucose) is stored in the body; in muscles, the liver and the brain.

Helicobacter pylori bacteria that cause inflammation and ulcers in the digestive tract.

Hiatus hernia a protrusion of part of the stomach upwards, through the diaphragm, so that digestive juices from the stomach are regurgitated into the oesophagus or gullet, causing damage to its lining and dyspepsia. (See gastro-oesophageal reflux disease.)

High-density (and low-density) lipoprotein (HDL and LDL) two forms of cholesterol that circulate in the blood. HDL, sometimes called 'good' cholesterol, lowers the risk of heart disease and helps balance the LDL, or 'bad' cholesterol, which increases the risk.

Human Genome Project the international research project to map the complete sequence of DNA that makes up human genes.

Hydrogenated (or partially hydrogenated) fats vegetable oils hardened by a chemical process that makes them into solid or semi-solid trans fatty acids (see below), widely used in commercial baking and for spreads, such as margarine.

Infarction death of living cells because of insufficient blood supply, frequently in the heart but other organs can be affected.

Insulin a hormone produced by the pancreas that helps the body absorb glucose (sugar) for energy.

Ischaemia   a deficiency of oxygenated blood flow to the tissues, usually because a blood vessel has become obstructed.

Ketosis   the process whereby the body draws upon glycogen stored in the tissues when the body has insufficient blood-sugar (glucose) to meet its energy needs – for example in the Atkins diet. Glycogen appears in the bloodstream as ketones, and makes the breath smell like pear-drops.

Leptin   a hormone produced in fat cells and in the lining of the stomach that communicates with the brain and is part of the body's weight-regulating system.

Liposuction   plastic surgery to remove localized fat under the skin using a suction pump.

Metabolic syndrome   a cluster of health problems that often occur together, including high blood-sugar, high blood pressure and a high level of fats in the blood, which can lead to cardiovascular disease, and which are often associated with excess fat around the abdomen.

Metabolism   the process by which cells in the body break down the constituents in food, absorb nutrients and dispose of waste.

Monounsaturated fat   a type of fat found in vegetables, like olive, walnut or rapeseed oil, and in some spreads. They have the same calorie content as other fats, but may protect against heart disease by lowering low-density lipoproteins (LDL, 'bad') levels without reducing HDL ('good') levels.

Neurotransmitters   naturally occurring chemicals that transmit messages to different parts of the brain and nervous system.

Obstructive sleep apnoea   a potentially fatal condition when someone snoring momentarily stops breathing while asleep.

Oedema   swelling of soft tissue caused by water and salt retention.

Omega-3 fatty acids   fats found principally in oily fish and some vegetable oils that may be protective against heart disease.

Opiates, also **opioid drugs**   naturally occurring or synthetically produced drugs that interrupt the message of pain before it is registered in the brain, producing euphoria. The body develops a tolerance to them and they are addictive.

Osteoarthritis   degeneration of the lining of the joints, usually but not always the result of wear and tear, leading to discomfort, loss of movement and enlargement.

Osteoporosis   loss of bone density leading to fragile, easily fractured bones.

Pancreas   an organ situated below the stomach which secretes digestive juices and hormones, including insulin.

Polyunsaturated fats   a type of fat derived chiefly from vegetables: corn, soybean, safflower and nuts; but also found in fish. These fats are liquid at room temperature and may be protective against heart disease.

Pre-eclampsia   a relatively common condition of late pregnancy characterized by high blood pressure, and protein in the urine (see proteinuria) and puffy ankles (see oedema), caused by abnormal kidney function. If not controlled can lead to eclampsia, involving convulsions, coma, miscarriage or even death.

Protein   the basic building blocks of all body structures, essential for the body to function and repair itself.

Proteinuria   when traces of a protein called albumin (like egg-white) are detected above a certain level in the urine, indicating potential kidney damage. It may be temporary, as in the later stages of pregnancy, or a warning sign of type 2 diabetes. Also known as albinuria.

Recessive or dominant (gene)   all genes are in pairs: one from each parent. A recessive gene paired with a dominant one will have the trait it controls suppressed. Only if identical recessive genes are paired will the trait they control for be expressed, affecting the way the organism develops.

Resistance training   exercise that uses the body's own weight to increase the load on muscles. Push-ups, squats, lunges and sit-ups are resistance training.

Saturated/polyunsaturated/monounsaturated fats   saturated fats are found mainly in animal products and some vegetables and are solid at room temperature. They have been found to raise cholesterol circulating in the blood. Unsaturated fats, which are liquid at room temperature, come mostly from fish, nuts or vegetables and are of two kinds: polyunsaturate – corn, sunflower and soybean oils – and monounsaturate – olive, nut and fish oils. These have a beneficial effect upon blood cholesterol.

Serotonin   a neurotransmitter (chemical messenger in the brain) that affects emotions, behaviour and thought.

Sphygmomanometer   device to measure blood pressure. The name comes from the Greek for 'pulse' (*sphygmus*) and for a device that measures things. It comprises a pressure-cuff wrapped round the arm that temporarily stops the flow of blood. As it is relaxed, the sound of the blood rushing back through the vessel can be heard with a stethoscope (see below). The pressure when the heart contracts is heard first and is called the systolic pressure. The lower pressure, driving the blood when the heart is at rest, is called the diastolic.

Stethoscope   a device that amplifies the sound of the heart beating and blood being driven through the different chambers and valves in the heart, enabling the skilled listener to detect abnormal function.

Synthesis   the body's manufacturing process.

Thyroid gland   a large gland located in the base of the neck which secretes a hormone that regulates body growth and metabolism.

Trans fats   (short for 'trans fatty acids') a form of saturated fat which occurs naturally and is produced artificially when oils are hydrogenated (see hydrogenated fats); considered harmful to health because, unlike the polyunsaturated oils from which they are derived, they limit the body's ability to regulate cholesterol.

Transactional analysis   a type of psychotherapy that uses the relationship (transactions) between patient and therapist to modify the patient's behaviour and attitudes towards others or his or her environment to modify behaviour or attitudes.

Vasoconstrictor/bronchodilator   drugs that act on the airways, prescribed to prevent an asthma attack. They 'constrict' blood vessels and 'dilate' the bronchial tubes.

VO2max   a crucial stage in exercise when the body can no longer increase the amount of oxygen it draws upon, even if the intensity of exercise increases. If the intensity of exercise increases further, the body starts to work *an*aerobically (without oxygen) and produces lactic acid which can be painful – sometimes referred to as 'the burn'.

Further reading

*Author recommendation

Barker, David, *Mothers, Babies and Health in Later Life*. Churchill Livingstone, London, 1998.

Calorie Counter. Collins Gems, London, 2006.

*Campos, Paul, *The Obesity Myth*. Gotham Press, New York, 2004.

Foster, Helen, *Eat 5*. Hamlyn, London, 2002.

Gaesser, Glenn, *Big Fat Lies: The Truth About Your Weight and Your Health*. Gurze Books, Carlsbad, Calif., 2002.

*Gard, Michael and Wright, Jan, *The Obesity Epidemic: Science, Morality and Ideology*. Routledge, London, 2005.

Hirschmann, Jane and Munter, Carol, *Overcoming Overeating: Conquer Your Obsession With Food*. Vermilion, London, 2000.

Humphries, Carolyn, *The Hugely Better Calorie Counter*. Foulsham, Slough, 2002.

*Hurst, Jan and Hubberstey, Sue, *Help Your Child Get Fit Not Fat*. Sheldon, London, 2005.

Kellow, Juliette and Walton, Rebecca, *The Calorie Carb and Fat Bible*. Weight Loss Resources, Peterborough, 2006: Tel. 01733 345592 for details or <www.weightlossresources.co.uk/diet/low_fat.htm>

Polivy, Janet and Herman, G. Peter, *Breaking the Diet Habit: The Natural Weight Alternative*. Basic Books, New York, 1983.

Riddoch, Chris and McKenna, Jim (eds), *Perspectives on Health and Exercise*. Palgrave Macmillan, London, 2002.

Robinson, Lynne, et al., *Official Body Control Pilates Manual: The Ultimate Guide to the Pilates Method – For Fitness, Health, Sport and at Work*. Macmillan, London, 2002.

*Vogel, Shawna, *The Skinny on Fat*. W. H. Freeman, Basingstoke, 1999.

Childhood obesity references in Chapter 5

Ebbeling, Cara B. et al., 'Childhood obesity: public-health crisis, common sense cure,' *The Lancet*, vol. 360, 10 August 2002.

Index

pauline frommer's

LAS VEGAS

spend less see more

2nd Edition

WITHDRAWN FROM STOCK

by Pauline Frommer
Shopping, gaming, and side trips by
Kate Silver

Series Editor: Pauline Frommer

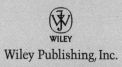

WILEY

Wiley Publishing, Inc.

Published by:

Wiley Publishing, Inc.

111 River St.
Hoboken, NJ 07030-5774

ISBN: 978-0-470-38528-9

Editor: Kathleen Warnock
Production Editor: Michael Brumitt
Cartographer: Guy Ruggiero
Photo Editor: Richard Fox
Interior Design: Lissa Auciello-Brogan
Production by Wiley Indianapolis Composition Services
Front and back cover photo © Lise Gagne/iStock Photo
Cover photo of Pauline Frommer by Janette Beckmann

For information on our other products and services or to obtain technical support,
please contact our Customer Care Department within the U.S. at 877/762-2974,
outside the U.S. at 317/572-3993 or fax 317/572-4002.

Wiley also publishes its books in a variety of electronic formats. Some content that
appears in print may not be available in electronic formats.

Manufactured in the United States of America

5   4   3   2   1